Music Therapy in Context

of related interest

Music for Life
Aspects for Creative Music Therapy with Adult Clients
Gary Ansdell
ISBN 978 1 85302 299 9

Music Therapy Research and Practice in Medicine
From Out of the Silence
David Aldridge
ISBN 978 1 85302 296 8

Music Therapy in Health and Education
Edited by Margaret Heal and Tony Wigram
Foreword by Anthony Storr
ISBN 978 1 85302 175 6

Music and People with Developmental Disabilities
Music Therapy, Remedial Music Making and Musical Activities
F. W. Schalkwijk
ISBN 978 1 85302 226 5

Grief and Powerlessness
Helping People Regain Control of their Lives
Ruth Bright
ISBN 978 1 85302 386 6

Making Music with the Young Child with Special Needs
A Guide for Parents
Elaine Streeter
ISBN 978 1 85302 960 8

Music Therapy in Context
Music, Meaning and Relationship

Mercedes Pavlicevic
Preface by Colwyn Trevarthen

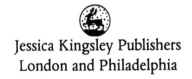

Jessica Kingsley Publishers
London and Philadelphia

Extract from *Lost in Translation* by Eva Hoffman. Copyright © Eva Hoffman 1989.
Used by permission of Dutton Signeta division of Penguin Books USA Inc.
and William Heinemann Ltd, UK.

Extract from *Miss Smilla's Feeling for Snow* by Peter Høeg, first published in Great Britain Harvill,
and in the USA by Farrer, Straus and Giroux in 1993. Copyright © Peter Høeg and
Munksgaard/Rosinante, Copenhagen 1992. English translation © Farrer, Straus and Giroux Inc
1993.
Reproduced by permission of Harvill Press.

Extract from *Under My Skin* by Doris Lessing. Copyright © Doris Lessing.
Reproduced by permission of HarperCollins Publishers, UK.

Figure from *The Art and Science of Music: A Handbook*, edited by Wigram, West and Saperston.
Copyright © Wigram, West and Saperston 1995.
Reproduced by permission of Harwood Academic Publishers, Switzerland.

First published in the United Kingdom in 1997
by Jessica Kingsley Publishers
116 Pentonville Road
London N1 9JB, UK
and
400 Market Street, Suite 400
Philadelphia, PA 19106, USA

Copyright © Mercedes Pavlicevic 1997
Preface copyright © Colwyn Trevarthen 1997

Printed digitally since 2010

Library of Congress Cataloging in Publication Data
A CIP catalogue record for this book is available from the Library of Congress

British Library Cataloguing in Publication Data
A CIP catalogue record for this book is available from the British Library

ISBN 978 1 85302 434 4

Contents

List of Figures

Acknowledgements

Several colleagues took the time and trouble to read through sections of the manuscript and gave me comments, criticisms and suggestions. I thank Ken Aigen in New York, Vanessa Richards in Johannesburg, and, in London, I thank Gary Ansdell, Sandra Brown, Sarah Caird, Jane Davidson, Jackie Robarts and Helen Tyler for their insights.

The support of others has been less directly but no less significantly, part of creating this book. Julienne Cartwright held the light for me a long time ago when the skies were dark and the winds cold and slow. Colwyn Trevarthen showed me how to sculpt my thoughts into words and on to paper. Philippa Kruger withstood mountains of files, scrap paper, short tempers and abstracted monologues during mealtimes. Thembani Lillian Miya tended to my well-being, while the ghost of my grandmother, Sophia Kazamin Symeonides, hovered unfailingly, reminding me that cleverness without imagination is barren egoism. Finally the gangsters and car-hijackers of Johannesburg have helped me to remember that life is precious: there is not too much of it to waste.

Special Notice

The identities of all the persons in the case studies have been changed to protect their privacy.

For my mother,
Iro Symeonides Pavlicevic
and in memory of my father,
Milovan Trifo Pavlicevic

Preface
A Theory for Therapy in a Different Voice

Music moves us because we move in musical ways – rhythmically, harmoniously, with gestures modulated in intensity, weight and resonance. And our rhythmical acts are linked in sequences that can be read as narratives or melodies. We are born like this. A paediatric neurologist can be trained to judge the health of a premature new-born infant's brain by evaluating the rhythms and grace of the spontaneous movements of the baby's limbs. Learning how to move better only confirms the authority of the inner 'conductor' in our minds. When forces in the body of a skilled athlete in full performance are measured, it is found that his or her movements are miraculously efficient. There is almost no waste energy or waste time. Body members and brain dance together with elegant precision, meeting environment with swing.

And this brings us to the natural connection between emotional and physical health, and the musicality of our moving. Ill health, affecting mind and body, interferes with the coherence, vitality and delicacy of our actions and gestures. The Norwegian musicologist, Jon-Roar Bjorkvold (1992) claims that the rhythm of our moving measures health at all stages of life, from before birth to old age. Acting poly-rhythmically, harmoniously and sympathetically in society expresses our vitality and sociable well-being. Robotic, disintegrated and anxious ways of behaving are both unmusical and unhealthy.

Yes, and above all, the tangible, visible and audible musicality of our behaviour communicates. It is as if we are caught in a social web of sound, made to sympathise and synchronise by the vibrations of threads that tug between us. We are born with the same motor time generators, tuning forks of the same key, which transfer energy between us with instantaneous sympathy. All human beings walk, breathe, gesture, speak within the same range of rhythms. These give the measure of time to our consciousness and memory, as well as to our actions. Variations in the impulses express emotions to which we are all sensitive. All attune to the changing mood that is expressed in changing tempos and harmony of behavioural expression.

These things are manifestly true. Why, then, do we have to work so hard to understand how a musical description can detect our sicknesses of mind and how musical treatment can heal them? Could it be that we become insensitive to fundamental motives? Are we missing part of the causes of our actions and our maladies? Is there a case for a new musical psychiatry?

Music therapist Mercedes Pavlicevic is a trained musician who uses her knowledge of musical form and expression and performing skill to help people strengthen their inner co-ordination of motives when it is disordered by illness and emotional distress. Mercedes has many years of experience in working with people who have lost musicality and fallen out of tune with others and their behaviours. She knows that sympathetically matched and directed musical communication can help a person feel more connected and happier, assisting him or her to function more sympathetically and more intelligently in their families and in society. Furthermore she has undertaken original research to determine what actually happens in music therapy sessions, and what changes over a series of sessions. I had the privilege of following this work and was impressed by how Mercedes could use her music therapy training to make an accurate and detailed analysis of the recorded performance of her patients and herself. I noted her demonstration that such analysis can serve as a sensitive diagnostic instrument, discriminating kinds of emotional illness and tracking improvements in the course of treatment.

What I learned from this research is the rich evidence of human expression that a skilled music therapist brings to light. There is a wonderful material for psychological interpretation here, and it is at quite a different level from the analysis that comes from study of language or from tests of cognitive function and problem-solving. The timing, quality of sound, phrasing and melodic narrative form of the performances recorded in music therapy sessions are so clearly information about the inner motives of the persons who made them. The recorded sound is rich in evidence of brain dynamics and their emotive features.

It is most unfortunate that, in our psychology, study of non-verbal communication is marginal. What has been called 'conversational analysis', in which cine films or video recordings are subjected to careful measurement and statistical analysis, has long been in possession of evidence that we humans interact with one another at great speed, synchronising with subtle rhythms of exchange. Our bodies express the impulses of our minds, and we react immediately to one another's expressions. Music makes this into sound that appeals directly to the inner sense of acting and feeling. This is a level of meaning where words may be superfluous. It is not good enough to call the communication 'non-verbal' as if it were a kind of darkness lacking the light of language. It deserves a better name.

But surely music is a product of culture, an artefact of training and the learning of rules of structure and interpretation. How can it have universal validity beyond the styles and traditions of the musical culture? Mercedes tackles this problem in an interesting way. She knows that music therapy training gives power of awareness and expression. After all, her musicianship is essential to her work, giving her rational control, analytic tools and a notation to keep a detailed record. But the essential music is there in its own right beneath the cultivated skills of description and execution. Completely untrained clients, admittedly skilled listeners, can join in the music creation and express themselves. Different 'foreign' musics are accessible to us. They can even be perceived to have their characteristic moods or personality, as if the genius of each culture leads it to explore one corner of human nature. Mercedes has lived and worked in South Africa, a mixed culture that has dozens of highly musical sources. She explains how a music therapist can dip into world music, now available in recordings as never before, as if into a palette of different colours. He or she can choose what tones best with the client's expressive and self-regulatory needs of the present.

I think the problem of meaning cannot be a simple one. There have to be two levels of meaning, at least. There is an explicit symbolic meaning that language can grasp and explain. And there is a more directly accessible meaning closer to the motives for acting and awareness. What holds these together in therapeutic work is emotion and the emotional narratives that make up the canvas on which the more detailed memories of our lives, our bodily selves and our companionships are painted. The battle between verbalising and rationalising practitioners of psychoanalysis and those who want to defend a more intuitive, spontaneous and personal dynamic closer to an active sense of what music is, can become bewildering and discouraging. We have to understand that these are legitimate ways of accessing the network of emotions that hold together consciousness, our sense of agency and our communication. That said, I have no doubt that music therapy has a more direct access to the critical processes at the core of human motivation, a core that language can never displace. Language has power over emotions, and it becomes the stuff of myths, elaborate arguments and theories and a great store of memories; but words, in speaking and in thinking, are added to a dynamic of acting and experiencing, and to the feelings that we give and receive in live conversation with other persons. The poetry and prosody of language, its expression, is at the core of its motivation and its communicability. Music translates this source directly.

There is something human about the messages and social celebrations of music that animals cannot share. Merlin Donald (1991) has identified a necessary first stage in the evolution of the human mind and culture that prepares the way to language, symbolic thought and all the modern paraphernalia of knowledge stored outside minds in cultural artefacts. He calls it *mimesis*, the ability to act, dance and sing out a narrative of experiences and feelings by moving the body, any part of it, with expressive rhythm, depicting absent events and imaginary transformations. With mimesis came the ability of humans to understand each others' acting as a dramatic, or melodramatic, message. This must be why, for modern humans, music always carries meaning beneath and beyond language.

I am sure this is the right theory because I have seen what power music has in communication with infants. Mothers' songs, action games and dances, and instrumental and recorded music of more popular 'folk' kinds, appeal to young infants many months before words have any sense, pleasing them, animating them and calming them to peaceful sleep. Infants also participate musically with skill. They hear music and they join in. We are certainly born musical. This musicality is an expression of the moods and self-regulations that infants and their companions, old and young, can share. It changes immediately with breakdown in affection, or if the infant is overcome with fear, sadness or anger.

Improvisational music therapy, as in the approach developed by Nordoff and Robbins, is a method of taking this ancient, inborn and life-long system of human motives in hand to help persons whose lives have lost coherence and companionship. It can bring joy by releasing the energy that is easily shared. It can control rage and lift despair. It deserves development to bring it into a legitimate central place in the range of treatments available in the mental health programme. It deserves innovative scientific research to validate its principles and procedures, and to relate these to the principles and procedures of other health professions, especially psychotherapies of all kinds, occupational therapies, and speech and communication therapies. Funding music therapy training will save money spent in treatments that are less responsive to patients' discordant motives, and therefore less effective. It is a fascinating application of human abilities, and we know too little about how it works.

Mercedes is one of a growing band of scientifically minded, musically dedicated therapists who are doing something about this. She wants to 'put music therapy on the map'. I think she has done a great job of explaining her wish in this book.

Colwyn Trevarthen
Emeritus Professor of Child Psychology and Psychobiology, University of Edinburgh
Fellow of the Royal Society of Edinburgh
Member of Norwegian Academy of Science and Letters

Introduction
In the Spirit of Copernicus[1]

Whenever I walk along the ground floor corridor at the Nordoff–Robbins Music Therapy Centre in London and find one closed door after another, I know that something is happening behind those closed doors: something to do with music, something private, spontaneous and unique to the persons on the other side.

Within the dimensions created and defined by the closed doors, music therapists, together with people of all ages and stages of life, are busy negotiating, developing and sustaining a therapeutic relationship through music. Although music therapists from diverse theoretical and practical backgrounds define distinctive therapeutic priorities, music is at the heart of all music therapy. It is the basis on which therapeutic relationships are created. It is also the basis on which, after the session, therapists (and clients) reflect not only about 'what happened' during the session, but 'what it means'.

It is the meaning of the musical-therapeutic act that this book explores. The musical event, in this instance, draws inspiration from the pioneering work of Paul Nordoff and Clive Robbins (1971, 1977), whose clinical improvisation techniques have become widely used, and known as Creative Music Therapy. Here, through the therapist and the client's spontaneous, joint improvisations on various tuned and untuned instruments – that may include drums, cymbals, metallophone, xylophone, marimba, guitar, piano, melodica, reed horns, zither and, that most personal and essential instrument of all, the human voice – a world of sound begins to take shape and fill the lives of the players: therapist and client(s). Through the spontaneous, joint musical act, therapist and client develop and extend a unique sense of themselves in relation to one another.

---

1   Ken Aigen's comments on sections of this work in progress helped me to formulate the ideas for this Introduction.

1

Although the act itself may be more or less recognisable as a musical activity, the act of generating its meaning is a complex, uncertain and, at times, highly unsatisfactory business that risks restricting, distorting and falsely enhancing the significance of the musical event. At the same time, of course, meaning can colour, nuance and greatly enrich what may sometimes feel like a rather bleak and undynamic event.

This book addresses some of the current music therapy debates to do with meaning, which may be summarised as follows. First, are words necessary in music therapy: do they enhance or detract from the musical-therapeutic act, from the legitimacy of music as a therapeutic medium? Second, since creative music therapy insists on the inherent therapy in music, and since music is an art form, can we be sure that clinical improvisation is distinct from 'pure' music improvisation? Third, if clinical improvisation is, indeed, distinct from music improvisation, what is the nature of this distinction? And fourth, how do music therapists address culture-specific nuances in music?

In these pages, meaning in music therapy is negotiated by revolving, and travelling between, various spheres of knowledge, selected for their potential support in this search (Chapter 1). Music therapy is, implicitly, at the heart of this search, and the reader looking for more explicit descriptions and information about the music therapy profession needs to consult existing literature (Ansdell 1995; Bruscia 1987; Bunt 1994; Heal and Wigram 1991; Nordoff and Robbins 1971, 1977; Priestley 1975).

Part 1 (Chapters 2 to 6) draws from the fields of music theory and music psychology, in order to explore meaning in music as art form, in contrast to music as therapy. This focus on musical meaning creates a resonance between music theorists and the various positions taken by music therapists, which range from asserting that therapy happens exclusively in the music created in clinical improvisation, to assertions that to think only in 'music' is therapeutically limited: words are essential for developing the full potential of music therapy meaning. Part 1 ends with explorations into the similarities and distinctions between music improvisation whose emphasis is musical, and clinical improvisation whose emphasis is inter-personal, thereby addressing the particular acuity that music therapists develop through training and practice.

Part 2 (Chapters 7 to 9) explores the relationship between music and human emotion, in order to establish why, and on what basis, music is used as a therapeutic agent. Here two perspectives are taken. In the first, some of the psychological literature on non-verbal communication is explored in order to clarify the inherent musicality of our communicative acts. The mirror is then turned the other way, to explore the nature of communicative emotion in the joint, spontaneous musical act generated in music therapy improvisation.

Part 3 (Chapters 10 to 12) draws concepts from psychodynamic theory into the music therapy sphere, in order to explore meaning, and verbal meaning in music therapy, from this very different perspective. Here the 'word and music' debate is refracted against psychodynamic concepts such as 'transference', 'counter-transference' and 'interpretation'. Each one of these realities clarifies and elicits meaning that is inherent in a relationship, whether it be musical, verbal or silent. The book ends by addressing the 'dark' side of being a therapist, challenging us to consider what it is that we, as therapists, seek, and why it is that we are drawn towards this work (Chapter 13).

In conclusion, it will be evident that these chapters offer no definitive meaning or single, argument-proof theoretical direction. Although much of the musing in these pages is based on clinical improvisation techniques, this book hopes to contribute to a broader music therapy discourse. Much meaning is yet to be uncovered, recovered and written, and a dialectic invitation such as this is open-ended. Rather than attempt to engage with all of the bodies of theory on which music therapists from all persuasions rely, only those bodies of theory that seem pertinent to this search are given prominence here. Some readers may find loud and irritating absences in this book and these may begin to define other firmaments to be explored.

After all, Copernicus moved on by thoroughly understanding, and moving on from, theories defined by Aristotle and Ptolemy – and, years later, his own shoulders supported Galileo's enquiries.

CHAPTER 1

Creating Meaning

Umuntu ungumuntu ngabantu
(Zulu: A human being becomes human through other human beings)

Constructing a Case Study

I am preparing for a public presentation on music therapy by watching a video recording of an individual music therapy session with 'Xolile', a ten-year-old child from an inner city Johannesburg slum. Xolile lives with his mother, a single parent who chars for a living, and he is a latchkey child, letting himself into the empty flat after school. Nobody knows whether, in fact, he does go home after school. He has been referred to music therapy because his teachers report him as being flat, difficult to reach, as having little feeling or regard for others, and as being a behavioural and an academic problem. They also report that there is little structure, guidance or nurture in his life. Xolile lives an isolated life.

The video that I am watching is of session 5. Xolile is subdued by the presence of the cameraman and soundman in the room. As I watch, I recall feeling guilty at the time of the session, for subjecting him to this stress, knowing that I want this material for archives, and knowing that this recording interferes with our therapeutic process: we are both 'on show'. Soon after this session, Xolile disappears from school. Payment of his school fees has been in arrears, and a tentative enquiry by the (sympathetic) school has resulted in him failing to show up, despite concerned and sustained attempts by the school to contact his mother.

In the video recording we are cross-legged, on the floor, with an alto-xylophone between us. On each side of the xylophone is an untuned percussion instrument: bongos to one side and split drum to the other. Xolile looks tense, his scarred face tight-lipped and his eyes lowered. He does not look at me throughout the seven-minute video excerpt, and sits uncomfortably on his feet, to try and hide the large hole in his socks. His clothes are grubby and he looks generally unhealthy.

I consult my notes of previous, untaped sessions, and read my record of an evolving familiarity with this child's tight energy. He initiates frequently in our spontaneous playing on various instruments that include xylophones, marimba, bongo drums, tambourine and reed horns. He does not imitate and 'follow' my playing, but prefers to 'do his own thing', creating sounds on the various instruments with gusto. But something is missing in our joint playing. In session 1, my notes describe him as, 'tough, a little man, strong, absolutely 'male'...his playing predictable and shaped enough for me to meet it...a feeling that he runs away with his playing...am not quite sure where I fit in'. In a later session, my notes report, '...fluctuating form in his playing, loud/soft, big/small', and in session 4, 'he took off on the bongos, hard fast playing: how do I meet this?'.

As I watch the video clip, I become aware that as Xolile and I take turns to create spontaneous sounds on the xylophone on the floor between us, we are a tightly knit dyad. There is a confluence between us, a rapid give and take, and the turn-taking is so smooth that if I close my eyes I cannot always tell who plays when. I notice that when I introduce any change to my playing, whether by playing a longer phrase, by slowing down or by doing something different, he ignores me. This does not mean that he does not respond to me: his response is to ignore me. I become aware of feeling controlled by him: he can do as he pleases, slipping in a change here, there, suddenly shortening his phrase, changing the metre – and I am there, responsive and supportive. This dynamic between us feels unbalanced in the sense of being unmutual: I am doing all the meeting in this interaction, and my own attempts at introducing variations in the music gain little reciprocity from him. And yet it does not feel as though he is avoiding contact with me.

There is something about this excerpt that I cannot quite crystallise in my mind, and this I need to do, especially for this public presentation. The sum of our playing is a good match of energy, congruence in our timbre and phrase lengths, the playing 'sounds good'. I ask myself why I am choosing this excerpt for case study material: is it to do with my feelings for him; with my loss at his sudden and unexplained disappearance?

Fitting different lenses

Viewed from the field of perceptual and/or cognitive music psychology, the video excerpt suggests that both child and therapist are neurologically intact. The players' perception of the pulse is established early in the improvisation; the perceptual grouping mechanisms appear to be negotiated smoothly and easily; the musical invariants are shared between them; and the improvisation reveals referents, suggesting that both players' musical memory is engaged throughout the seven-minute excerpt.

Viewed from social music psychology, the cross-cultural scenario is in focus. The therapist is European, has a traditional Western classical training in music, and the child is African. Their cultures are worlds apart, and sub-Saharan African culture does not separate music from 'life'. Where does this Western music therapy fit within the African context of music, healing and ritual? Where does his Africanness correspond to the Western model of therapy?

The ethnomusicologist might detect that the therapist hasn't quite got the sub-Saharan African feel for the music: her playing is subtly flatter and 'squarer' than his. Is the child compromising his African musicianship in order to play with the therapist?

A music theorist watching this clip might enquire about the meaning and associations of the music for each of the players, thinking of meaning as being universal or culturally specific, and where the divergent sets of meanings coincide. The focus of enquiry might include how the musical structure of this improvisation might best be described.

A behavioural psychologist would report that the child is co-operating with the therapist and, although his posture is slightly tense and uncomfortable, he is obviously engaged in the session. How does this correspond to his behaviour in the classroom: does he need more one-to-one attention, can the classroom provide the affirmation that he is receiving in music therapy, could attending music therapy sessions be used as a reward for good behaviour?

Finally, a psychotherapist might ponder the meaning of the tautness of the therapist–child relationship, and reflect on how serious, un-light, un-soft it is. Where is this child's playfulness? The therapist reports something missing: there is external or structural interplay, so something about them is bonded. But a 'feeling' is missing. Is this how the child experiences the world – he can 'perform' well, go through the motions of living, but there is a deadness inside him which the therapist, in counter-transference, experiences? She reports feeling controlled by him: does he need to 'be in control'? How does this relate to his early relationships, to his current lifestyle, to what is happening between therapist and child? What about the choice of this material for a public presentation: is it a reflection of the nature of the therapist's counter-transference with this particular child?

Creating perspectives

Each of these 'lenses' offers different perspectives on the video clip, and none of them is especially alien to the music therapist. Each set of meanings reflects a particular body of knowledge, which potentially enriches the discipline of music therapy, and each is, I believe, enriched by 'looking at' music therapy (Figure 1.1). At the same time, taken in isolation, none of these lenses quite 'fits' with the experience of music therapy.

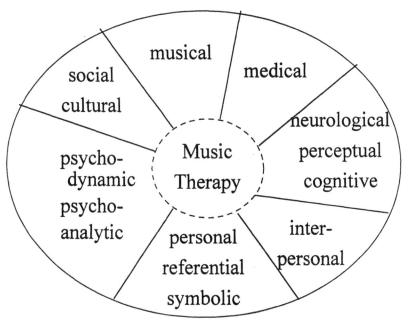

Figure 1.1 The meanings that we may assign to, and derive from, music therapy practice

What does the discipline of music therapy 'do' with perspectives from allied fields? It seems that as music therapists, we range in extremes from a position that refuses to import theories and meanings from other fields, preferring the 'pure' phenomenon of music therapy – whatever that means. At the other extreme is the position that borrows liberally – and not always convincingly – from other theoretical frameworks, in describing music therapy, in theorising about it and in reporting on sessions.

In examining the different ways that music therapists 'speak about' their work, we find a range of discourses, and each discourse frames the work within a particular set of meanings. Throughout this book, the word 'discourse' is used loosely to describe a set of meanings conveyed by language, as well as the relationship between language and the event. This relationship may be very close or very obtuse. Language may explain the event, describe it; language may construct the way that we see the event, and it may begin to operate independently of the event, becoming a discourse that is self-perpetuating, and that may be analysed as 'social text' through 'discourse analysis'.

Music Therapists Speak: Choosing a Discourse

Kay Sobey (1992, p.20) suggests that music is a 'short-cut to the unconscious', undermining defences and touching us suddenly and deeply, while Elaine Streeter (1987), sees music as reflecting current feelings, creating defences and re-enacting earlier patterns of relating. Each of these statements uses language that makes assumptions about our familiarity with psychodynamic theory: concepts such as 'the unconscious' and 'defences'.

Alyson Carter (1992) uses Jungian-based language when she states that music is a bridge between the ego – the temporal, material, day-to-day, outer – and the psyche – the inner, lasting. Robin Howat (1992), too, uses Jungian analytic concepts when he suggests that the language of music expresses directly the unconscious, the archetypal and the imaginary. None of these descriptions, however, gives us a clear picture of how these thoughts came about.

Jackie Robarts' (1994) comments are more philosophical and less grounded in a specific theoretical approach when she states: 'The paradoxes of our deepest sensibilities, which seem to lie beyond the grasp of the intellect, assume a particular significance in the music therapy process: spirit and matter, time and space, inner and outer reality – not dualities, but two aspects of human experiencing, held in perpetual dynamic interplay' (p.230).

But what is the effect of these various languages on the audience? Is there a risk that music therapists make assumptions about concepts and meaning with those who may be from the verges of another discipline? Can music therapists comfortably assume an understanding as to how these 'borrowed' concepts fit with music therapy practice, simply because the 'borrowed' language seems appropriate?

For example, what does it really mean, when Robin Howat (1992) discusses music as expressing the unconscious? If I were a Freudian, my understanding of the unconscious would be rather different from someone who is a Jungian analyst, and this again would differ from a cognitive psychologist, a Rogerian counsellor, and so on. One effect of borrowing language, is that it 'packages' the music therapy experience for us. Perhaps a little too neatly. It saves us the trouble of first checking the packaging.

Another consideration is the effect of these discourses on the practice of music therapy. Here Ken Aigen (1991) cautions against attempting to 'fit' music therapy practice into a set of rules, whether these be medical, psychological, political or whatever, as this risks compromising and diminishing the complexity of the practice. In other words, theory and theoretical frameworks ought not to 'prescribe' music therapy practice, telling music therapists how to think and how to tailor their practice. However, it seems that these theoretical discourses can usefully 'describe' the practice, enabling the descriptions to shift from a purely descriptive level of reporting and encompass a broader spectrum of thought.

There is, indisputably, a plus to borrowing language, meaning or theories from allied paradigms. In doing so a common area is defined between music therapy and other professions. Phrases such as 'the unconscious', 'defences' and 'the ego', are not exclusive to Jungian or Freudian psychoanalysts, or to music therapists. In using terms such as these, music therapists may be choosing not to seal and mystify their work, but to negotiate an area of meaning within which various disciplines contribute – and draw inspiration. And perhaps this is the primary value of using – or rather, creating – a common language, as endorsed by Aldridge, Brandt and Wohler (1990), rather than creating our own discourse, a discourse that is separate, indigenous to music therapy and potentially available exclusively to music therapists.

Rather than create a dialectic between these two positions, i.e. on the one hand 'refusing to borrow' and on the other 'borrowing liberally', it seems that a balance between them needs to be struck: a position that states that, rather than arguing for and against theory being 'music therapy theory', the essential is for theory to be loyal to practice, to be genuine in its participation with practice, to ensure that theory and meaning are *close* to practice, rather than distant from it. Theory explains, and at times interprets, practice, but it needs to be closely and dynamically related to, and inspired by, practice. It seems that if theory and practice become too distanced from one another, we are left with a practice that is impoverished in terms of meaning and a theory that withers away from its source.

But let us pause for a moment and consider whether, in fact, in creating meaning we want to use words at all. Can meaning remain in the musical? Is the musical-therapeutic experience really 'itself' – does this suffice in terms of its meaning?

To Speak or to Sound?

In her editorial for the *Journal of British Music Therapy*, Helen Odell (1989) quotes from Reik, who suggests that the act of formulating an idea (whether a feeling, a hunch or an image) into words renders it less likely to slip away into our unconscious. Thoughts that are not formulated verbally, Reik suggests, cannot resist withdrawing and being repressed. We 'lose' them: they can once again harbour in our unconscious and, presumably, play havoc with our lives.

In terms of meaning, does this suggest that an idea that is embodied in sound or music is less powerful or less significant than one embodied in words? Is it only through words that real awareness of meaning and consciousness occurs?

I think that it is fairly safe to assume that Reik was unaware at the time (1949) of the possibilities of music therapy. My own understanding is that once a thought (for want of a better word) is expressed or embodied, *no matter what the medium of expression*, it has a new 'power'. The act of embodying, or of making the thought 'flesh', be it through music, sculpture, art or words, prevents it from being suppressed, repressed or disappearing altogether. However, the nature of this embodiment may give the thought a different emphasis, a different dynamism and a different colour.

What happens, then, when we speak about music therapy – about the musical act? Do words help us to capture the experience more essentially? Does 'speaking about' it prevent the experience from evaporating, receding, deserting us? When working with verbal clients, is it through verbalising the musical, non-verbal act that both the therapist and the client give the experience meaning – and possibly prevent it from slipping away or disappearing? Were we to leave the musical experience to speak for itself, would it remain unconscious, un-recovered, unaccessed by the client? Would this be limiting to a client who was fully verbal – or would it enhance the experience? Might the act of speaking detract from the power of the experience itself? Would it not impose a constricting order? Push it this way or that? Or, as Chris Gale (1992) puts it, do words potentially freeze ideas into coherence and consistency?

Why is it that, as is evidenced by this book, we feel the need to conceptualise the event verbally? Why do we write about music therapy?

The word in crisis

George Steiner (1985) alerts us to the crisis of language-based concepts and understanding that faces the 20th century. Our world has become saturated by words to a such degree that the association between (verbal) language and 'reality' is in question. This redefinition of the association is not just a linguistic crisis, involving linguistic scholars, but one that affects all disciplines, including philosophy and psychology. Steiner suggests that we are currently in a 'post-verbal' civilisation: one in which the word is 'in retreat'. The word is losing its power. One of the consequences of the long dominance of 'the word', is that our senses have become narrowed. We face not just a linguistic crisis, but a crisis of the senses; we seem unable simply to experience; we need to 'talk about' in order to 'create' and to 'test' reality.

It seems as though, as creative arts therapists, music therapists are uniquely and powerfully placed to give primacy to the senses. And yet despite our therapeutic focus on the non-verbal musical event, it seems that our explicitly verbal and 'reasoning' cultures beguile us towards the word. We seem to feel that unless we can talk about the musical experience, then (1) the non-verbal experience is incomplete; (2) professional colleagues will think that we do not know what we are doing; and (3) our clinical grasp of the work will be questioned – we might be seen to be doing 'just music'.

There seems, then, to be a paradox. On the one hand there is the strength of music as a non-verbal, therapeutic event and, at the same time, a pull towards using words to convey and portray the musical act. Certainly, current debate among music therapists suggests that the question of 'verbalising' has generated a crisis in music therapy thinking.

In some instances, music therapists question the validity of using words at all. The Nordoff–Robbins approach to music therapy, in particular, has traditionally been understood and interpreted as focusing on the musical event and bypassing words. All very well when working with non-verbal clients, as, indeed, Nordoff and Robbins did, but what if the client decides to talk? To talk about the music, to talk about his or her life, to engage in a verbal, as well as a musical, relationship?

When Colin Lee (1992) asks whether words are a useful paradigm to explain or evaluate music therapy sessions, since words come from such a totally different source to music, he is referring to 'talking about' the work. The title of Leslie Bunt's book, *Music Therapy: An Art Beyond Words* (1994), suggests that words might not get to the 'beyond' that is elicited in music therapy practice. Robin Howat (1992) suggests that the musical experience transcends any symbolic (verbal) attachment and/or interpretation that we may wish to bring in addition – we do not need words.

Ken Aigen (1991) too cautions against the use of words, in particular words from a discipline such as psychotherapy. He suggests that musically coded thought has its own value, and that verbally encoded thought is not the only knowledge. Verbal renditions, he suggests, must be accountable to the legitimacy – and primacy – of musical thought.

It seems, then, that one of the arguments presented against the use of words in sessions is that words may corrupt the 'purity' or 'integrity' of the musical experience. Moreover, music therapists who use words in sessions are often perceived as working 'psychodynamically', rather than purely *music*-therapeutically, and this bias is seen as compromising the validity of the musical act.

In one sense, the confounding of words with psychodynamic stance is not altogether surprising, given that, like (verbally based) psychotherapy practice, much that goes on in music therapy is beyond: beyond words or beyond music. And both music therapists and psychotherapists use words in describing and thinking about this 'beyondness'. This 'beyond' can be seen as the movements and shifts within the patient, within the therapist and between the therapist and patient. Psychotherapists resonate with these qualities through words and, at the same time, beyond the spoken words, listening to the client's movement, gestures, postures and intonation – as well as to the complex layers of meaning of the words themselves. In music therapy, clinical improvisation elicits these shifts, this 'beyondness' instantly, through the quality of interlocking of the musical impulses of the therapist and client. Music therapists, who often do not use words at all and whose work with severely disabled people may prevent access to verbal language, resonate with the client's investment of themselves through the musical act. This act cannot move towards concrete, referential meaning (where a spade is a spade), as can words.

Gary Ansdell (1995) suggests that the musical experience in music therapy is itself the phenomenon ('the map is not the territory'), it does not require verbal explanation or interpretation. He crystallises the gap between words and music with the idea of the 'music therapists' dilemma', drawn from Charles Seeger, who, as an ethnomusicologist, faced the gap. However, while the phenomenon is undoubtedly powerful and direct, the 'map' that portrays the phenomenon adds a breadth of meaning that being on the territory cannot provide. Again, rather than polarise the 'map' and the 'territory', a position that acknowledges the value of both the territory and the map – in tandem with one another – seems more attractive and enriching.

There is an inherent difficulty in using one form of language to describe and capture something that is qualitatively and conceptually distinct from it. In contrast to music, which is synchronous, multi-levelled and spatial, speech language has the choice of being linear and sequential, temporal in a narrow sense. Can words really describe music? When the composer Karlheinz

Stockhausen was asked this question, he responded with an absurd description of how a piece of music described a tree (Cott 1974). The absurdity was in the words that he used, which made absolute nonsense of the idea. However, Stockhausen's prank raises the question as to whether music can describe – or portray – verbal ideas. Leaving aside the use of words in songs, and the arguments of music theorists, there is a point to be made here with regard to words and theory being used to prescribe music therapy practice. The act of clinical improvisation is spontaneous, unpredictable and endlessly surprising: to make this fit into a theoretical framework is to risk diminishing it.

Marion Milner's (1957) comments about trying to capture the essence of a work of art through words are apposite here. She talks about the false certainty, the deceptive sanity that can be imposed on a drawing that may appear chaotic (p.76): as soon as the drawing becomes 'recognised' by the intellect, its rhythm becomes suddenly pushed to one or other direction. She also distinguishes between thinking in the private language of one's imagination and the more public thinking that takes place through shared language. James Hillman (1975), too, suggests that confronting images – talking, describing, unravelling them – can prejudice and subvert the imagination into the control of mind, knowledge and strength, at the expense of freer imaginings.

All of these issues apply to the way that we make sense of music therapy. For instance, words can move along a spectrum from being highly descriptive and concrete about the actual event, towards being abstract, weak on description and metaphorical. Theory can move along a spectrum from being rigorous and systematic, close to music therapy practice, to being weak and distant from practice (Figure 1.2). Each of these four polarities, when taken as an entity, is unsatisfactory and potentially hermetically sealed. Thus graphic descriptions ((d) in Figure 1.2 such as, client played this and then therapist did that and then client did this and then that, etc.) may leave the audience wondering what 'doing this and that' means, especially when the description is weak on theory. Similarly a presentation that is rigorously theoretical, but weak on description (b), while entertaining our sophist tendencies, may leave us unclear about the basis – both clinical and the musical – for these ideas. Talk that is weak on theory and abstract in description (c), we hope to abandon altogether. The ideal seems to be a dialectic (both/and) between description and theory, positioned at (a), rather than treating theory and description as a duality (either/or).

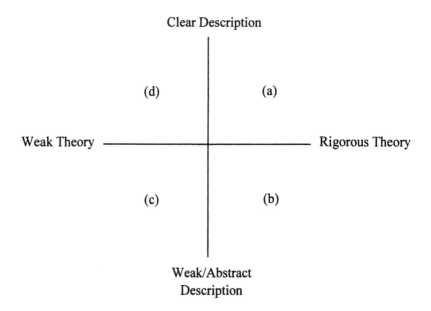

Clear Description

(d)   (a)

Weak Theory ———————————————— Rigorous Theory

(c)   (b)

Weak/Abstract
Description

Figure 1.2 Relationship between music therapy theory and description of clinical work

So, do we speak or do we not speak? Does music therapy need words or should we stop talking and 'get on with it' – just do it?

Music therapist Kay Sobey (1992) reminds us that the use of verbal language can blunt our capacity to relate directly to feelings. The directness of the musical act heightens our sensitivities to the feeling of life – especially when working with those who have poor language, communication or expressive skills. This sane reminder jolts us into a critical reality: that the needs of clients and patients are paramount, and that in theorising and speaking about the work, we owe them – and our work with them – an integrity that is beyond sophistry and intellectualisation.

The last word goes to Chris Gale (1992) who states:

> When arguments are advanced for the strict adherence to a 'musical model' is it really intended that all considerations other than the actual succession of notes be disregarded?...surely the expressive needs of clients should determine the shape and boundaries of sessions, rather than any particular 'model' which may mean little from the client's viewpoint...if our work is concerned with wholeness then we should not compartmentalise in this way. After all, music is there to broaden possibilities, not to restrict them (p.26).

Testing Reality

Everyone, at some time or other, needs to 'test reality': how does my thought 'sound' when I tell you about it? How does my thought 'feel' when I listen to, and look at, your listening and your response to what I say? And how does my 'feeling' change my thinking? Africans of Southern Africa talk of *ubuntu*: it is through you that I know I exist; you help me to define my reality. The philosopher Hegel alerted us to becoming fully ourselves through being recognised by another, and recognising this recognition.

The practice of music therapy has an 'internal' reality which is intimate, vibrant and fluid. When I talk with others who share this reality, our conversations make huge assumptions, and to outsiders conversations may appear odd and stilted – in the same way that conversation between intimate couples is incoherent to others and exclusive. However, music therapy exists in the world that includes psychologists, psychiatrists, psychotherapists, doctors, parents and teachers of disabled children, speech therapists, social workers and neurologists, some of whom share underlying premises about the role and meaning of music therapy. In talking 'about', we can make no assumptions about how others hear what we say. In dialogues with those who are theoretically distanced from music therapy, part of the dialogue itself consists of tackling words and grappling with concepts, in order to develop meaning about the work that both parties can share. This negotiation of meaning needs to take place at the descriptive level, as well as at the level of inference and interpretation.

The Limits of Understanding

This book explores, creates and negotiates music therapy meaning in relation to theory, and theory uses words. Once music therapists enter into verbal language and thought, we distance ourselves from the essence of the experience of being-in-music. In a sense, even our personal, interior verbal monologues about music therapy are a form of 'reality testing' for the actual musical experience. The risk in using words publicly is that we may be lulled, despite our instincts, towards another kind of reason, order, logic. In dialoguing with disciplines that have differently evolved models and framework, we may be judged cruelly because we speak a different kind of logic. We may be dismissed as being metaphysical or poetic or, at least, unsystematic. Verbal thought, thanks to the 'Enlightened' past 400 years, is not altogether patient with incoherence and disorder – for not only does this belong to the fanciful world of poetry, but it is also trespassing into madness. And madness, as we have learnt (often to our detriment), is not 'reality'.

The main concern of this book is to examine the meanings that different discourses may not only create, but help to propagate about music therapy and in music therapy. Meaning is not a set of fixed concepts, but rather a dynamic and fluid weave. However, a set of meanings does not necessarily fit together neatly like a jigsaw puzzle, but different meanings may chaff against each other. These potential conflicts, I believe, add immense richness to meaning, and in this sense this book does not attempt a (cosy) synthesis, but rather chooses to nudge, prod, challenge and cross-examine. Moreover, music therapy practice is complex, multi-faceted, not always logical or linear, and it generates meaning that is not just subjective or objective, but also intersubjective. Meaning continues to be sculpted by 'engaging with' and 'being engaged with' other sets of meanings.

Theorists (and meta-theorists, who theorise theory itself) often interpret and describe events from the outside, creating meaning that risks being too objective, separate from a reality that is treated as passive. For a practising music therapist this position is not only impossible, but would be inauthentic. The work – my session with Xolile – is not separate from my reading of any theory or text, and the clinical work colours the meaning that I derive from reading theory. Thus in reading a text on music therapy, a client might come to mind, reminding me of what I am reading and infusing the text with colour and aliveness. At the same time, during the process of writing or thinking, various aspects of sessions appear, to shed clarity – and to infuse a dynamism – on my thoughts.

This book, therefore, does not turn its back on those professions with 'uncomfortable' discourses but chooses to enter into dialogue with them, in order to broaden the 'interpretative repertoire' (Potter and Wetherell, cited in Banister *et al.* 1994, p.94) that music therapy might develop. By broadening the palette of meaning, it seems that we can only enrich our understanding of music therapy practice and thought. I therefore refute the argument that music therapy theory cannot import from other discourses, on the grounds that by doing so, music therapy risks compromising its uniqueness and indigenous character. Also I disagree with the argument that since psychotherapy is predominantly verbal (which I question), and music therapy is essentially non-verbal, importing psychotherapy concepts is inappropriate. However, I accept that music therapy theory needs to be grounded in practice, since it is the live, here-and-now experience that energises and inspires our thinking. I believe that theory *must* be useful to practice, rather than being, and becoming, self-important, clever, inaccessible and creating its own paradigms and horizons.

PART I

CHAPTER 2

Music, Meaning and Music Therapy
A View from Music Theory[1]

I am in the middle of an improvisation with Noel, an artist who has come for six music therapy sessions to help him to 'loosen up'. Noel is surrounded by the temple blocks, bass and conga drums, two cymbals and bongos, as well as marimba and xylophone. His playing is busy, rapid and 'tight', and my own spontaneous playing at the piano meets and reflects his 'tight busy-ness'. I listen to his ongoing rhythmic play, his small melodies, made up mostly of adjacent notes on the marimba, going up and down, up and down. I listen for change. For three sessions we have been playing this tight busy-ness, and my musical and interactive expectations are all but hypnotised. I am aware of being almost bored, not quite paying attention, keeping track of what he is doing on 'automatic pilot'. My earlier attempts at changing, extending, altering propelled his playing into chaos and disorder, and I have decided to 'sit tight' musically, for the time being, and wait.

Something changes. He extends the (monotonous) rhythm, and at the same time he does an interval leap instead of the preceding adjacent notes. My attention is caught: something 'meaningful' is happening. I not only think it, I feel it. I have a flush of excitement, because even though I have been waiting, what Noel does is unexpected, and our joint, spontaneous playing can begin to move on. My change in level of arousal is triggered by something within the music – it has to do with the change of rhythm, the melodic leap, and the succeeding gradual build-up in intensity.

Meaning in Music: A View from Music Theory

The question of meaning in music is a vast issue that straddles many disciplines, including those of philosophy, psychology, semiotics, linguistics and acoustics, and it seems that there is undying enthusiasm for exploring

---

1   I am grateful to Gary Ansdell for his comments on this and the following chapter.

why and how music is meaningful to human beings; why it is such a powerful personal and social phenomenon; and why we use it as a therapeutic tool. This chapter explores 'how music means' for music therapy practice, and the emphasis here is on the *musical* meaning, rather than on the therapeutic/psychological/interactive. In terms of dipping into other discourses, the main 'dip' is semiotics, the study of signs, although this discussion does not pretend to address or present an overview of semiotics. This parallel theory offers insights to do with meaning, and these are hauled in, so to speak, to explore meaning in music therapy, and to challenge and extend some concepts in music therapy practice and theory.

Jean-Jaques Nattiez, the Canadian semiotician, opens his famous book, *Music and Discourse* (1990), with the following statement:

> This book is based upon a hypothesis that I shall immediately state: the musical work is not merely what we used to call the 'text'; it is not merely a whole composed of 'structures' (I prefer in any case, to write of 'configurations'). Rather, the work is also constituted by the procedures that have engendered it (acts of composition), and the procedures to which it gives rise: acts of interpretation and perception (p.ix).

Nattiez' statement alerts us to one of the problems that prevail in existing discussions on musical meaning, that is, that 'music' is usually thought of in rather narrow terms and, more specifically, as being listened to and therefore being separate from the subject who is listening. In this context the listener has nothing to do with the acts of composition, re-creation and interpretation of the score. Even though some music therapists do indeed listen to pre-composed music as part of their work (for example, those who practise Helen Bonny's Guided Imagery in Music (Bonny 1978a, 1978b)), the tenor of this discussion is not only for their benefit. Musical meaning is the subject of ongoing debate and strong feelings, and some points from this debate may well challenge how music therapists 'mean'. Those who improvise music in their sessions and who, like Nattiez, think of music as a multi-faceted event made up of creating the musical work, while at the same time listening to it and interpreting it, are faced with multiple meanings that impinge on one another.

Absolutely no references: the absolutist position

One of the primary distinctions that emerges in the literature on musical meaning is the well-debated distinction between musical meaning being *absolute* and *referential*. Carl Dalhaus' essay on 'absolute music' (1989) reminds us that the argument can be traced back to the Middle Ages, when those who supported 'pure' music derided those who supported the use of words in a composition: the written text would detract from the 'pure' meaning of the music itself. Pure music was embodied in instrumental music, which was seen as the most sublime form of music, allowing a quasi-religious experience of listening. This music had no distracting text or extra-musical references to sully it; it was the supreme art, and its subjectivity was, simply, itself. I am not sure what the 'absolutists' would have made of music therapy, where music portrays something other than just itself and, in some instances, may be interpreted as referring to some event, person, or act in a person's life.

Many centuries and historical developments have punctuated the years between then and now, and although the distinction has become somewhat gentler, those in the absolutist camp suggest that meaning in music is intrinsic to the music itself. Here the meaning is inherent in the formal aspect of the music, i.e. it is what the rhythm, melody, harmony 'do' among themselves that makes the music meaningful to the listener. The absolutist view was supported by Stravinsky, who made his position clear in his famous Harvard lectures (1970). Meaning, for Stravinsky, is only musical. Music cannot express feelings, emotions or, for that matter, anything that is non-musical. As well as being absolutist, Stravinsky's position is what Leonard Meyer (1956, 1967) has called the 'formalist' viewpoint, in the sense that the purely musical meaning is primarily intellectually based. The meaning lies in the intellectual recognition of formal changes.

Eduard Hanslick, in his work entitled *The Beautiful in Music* (1957) takes an absolutist position, stating that: 'Definite feelings and emotions are unsusceptible of being embodied in music' (p.24). In other words, music cannot portray or embody feelings or emotions. However, he does acknowledge that, rather than the feelings themselves, the 'qualities' of feelings (such as 'whisperings' and 'stormings') can be reproduced in music – and this somewhat confused his position as an absolutist.

When Hanslick advocates that music contains 'whisperings and stormings', he suggests that the forms of music portray something that is not only musical, unlike Stravinsky who proposes that musical forms are only musical forms. Although Hanslick is an absolutist, his position is also an 'expressionist' one. This means, as Nattiez reminds us, that music may well be expressive of feeling-forms, but these feeling-forms are contained within the music itself. Thus, according to Hanslick, music may well express the qualities of sorrow or joy, but these feelings are in the music (rather than in the listener).

For the absolutists, the meaning is 'absolutely' in the music and nowhere else: it is not within the listener and it is not to do with anything other than the music, which the listener recognises, and then derives and assigns meaning to this recognition (Figure 2.1).

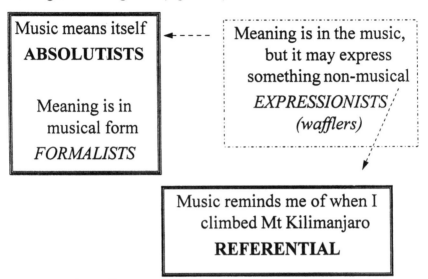

Figure 2.1 What and how music means

Referring to music: the referentialist position

In contrast to the absolutist camp are the 'referentialists', who believe that the meaning of music is to do with its context and associations, rather than just with the music itself. Here the listener brings something else, something non-musical, to the musical experience, and this act renders the music meaningful to the listener. This may mean that in listening to a piece of music we experience the feelings we had when hearing the piece in the past. For example, the first movement of Shostakovitch's first symphony always reminds me of the excruciating heat I once experienced during a solitary weekend in the Magaliesberg Mountains north of Johannesburg. This association is triggered by the context of listening, and its meaning is personal and rather idiosyncratic, having little to do with the music itself.

Referential meaning, however, is not only personal: it may also have to do with culture: in certain cultures, certain musics and musical events have specific, non-musical meanings. John Blacking's (1973, 1987, 1995) 'social' view of music suggests that musical meaning is contextual: music cannot be separated from its relationship to, and role in, society. He feels that music for music's sake does not exist, and that all music is, in a sense, *folk* music. Blacking says, explicitly, that the patterns in music represent the patterns of organisation within a society: how people relate to one another, how hierarchies are created and acknowledged, and how people interact. For example, for the Venda, as for other sub-Saharan cultures, all people are considered to be musical, and all partake actively in the musical rituals of the culture. Furthermore, Blacking (1987) reminds us that for sub-Saharan people, '…activities which might be described as ritual, aesthetic, or artistic, are seen *not* merely as part of the superstructure of human social life, but as fundamental to intellectual and social life, and as integral parts of the process of production' (p.25). He goes on to say that for many African people, musical communication and the bodily experiences of the music are linked to other experiences and ideas. Music itself has no power, says Blacking. Moreover, not only is music about the community but it also helps to embody and define the relationship between the individual and their community. Indeed African music can reveal how a group of people are organising and involving themselves in their own communal relationships (Chernoff 1979). Here it would seem that music not only tells us about itself, but it can, in addition, tell us about something else – point towards something other than itself in a specific way.

This ethnomusicology perspective is a very different view from the absolutists of the 'Ancients' camp, who would turn in their graves at the suggestion that music has no meaning as itself, apart from its particular social and cultural context. This view has been expanded upon more recently by those ethnomusicologists who suggest that music does not simply reflect culture but is instrumental in negotiating hierarchies within a culture, transforming social space and identifying boundaries between social groups (Stokes 1994).

While much of these discussions sounds highly theoretical and somewhat spurious to clinicians, there is something of value for music therapists, in the sense of us clarifying for ourselves how we come to assign meaning to music in music therapy practice.

Information theory

Leonard Meyer (1956, 1967) uses different terms to approach the question of referential and absolutist meaning in music, distinguishing between what he calls 'designative' meaning and 'embodied' meaning in music. Where music refers to, or indicates something, that is *unlike* itself, it gives rise to designative meaning. Where the music indicates something that is like itself in kind, then Meyer talks about 'embodied' meaning. This is not quite the same as the absolutist position (that says that the meaning is exclusively within the music and exclusively musical), but is close to it (the meaning is *like* the music) in the sense that it is the form of the music that needs to be recognised as being present in the embodied object.

Meyer, being more pragmatic than the Ancients and the Modernes, suggests that music can give rise to both kinds of meaning. It can evoke associations and connotations for the listener, and these may come from the listener's own life experiences. However, at the same time, music can evoke its own meaning for the listener, by creating expectations of subsequent events in the music itself. What is known as Meyer's 'information theory' fits here – i.e. within 'embodied' meaning. Meyer suggests that meaning remains 'neutral' when we can take for granted the direction of a piece of music – in his terms, the musical stimulus is habitual: it is an 'unthinking' stimulus. Musical meaning is the result of a delay or block of our expectant habits, or the result of ambiguity in the music, or of something unexpected happening. All of these produce uncertainty in the listener: it is the interruption, variation or inhibition of these expectations that results in a heightened state of arousal, and this heightened state, which Meyer considers to be an emotional state, renders the music meaningful for the listener.

Meyer's information theory preceded the work of cognitive music psychologists who, as we shall see later, suggest that it is our own apprehension of musical structure and musical events that renders music meaningful.

Musical Meaning and Music Therapy

Music therapists (many of whom create music in sessions) need to bear in mind that the above discussions are based on 'listening' to music. This implies that the listener and the music are separate entities – i.e., the listener has nothing to do with the creation or performing of the music. However, the discussions alert us to the different ways of listening to music, all of which are pertinent to music therapists. Nicholas Cook (1990, 1994) describes the different ways of listening to music, and addresses the supposed distinction between how musicians and non-musicians listen to music. In listening to a musical work, musicians may perceive its formal structure, noting the performer's techniques, the orchestral and instrumental colour, and so on. This 'musicological' listening colours the nature of experiencing music. However, non-musicians, tend to respond directly (and non-intellectually) to the sound itself, and derive direct pleasure from the music, without necessarily 'understanding' it. Another mode of listening – which may be part of musicological and non-musicological listening – is to create images triggered by the sound – a piece of music may remind us of a walk in a beautiful autumn wood, a bleak grey wet winter's day, or a delicious love affair. This is close to the referentialist position. In music therapy, we ask ourselves how the therapist and client listen, and what meaning is assigned to what they hear.

For example, music therapists using the Bonny method of Guided Imagery in Music (Bonny 1978a, 1978b) invite clients to listen to pre-composed music while imagining a context that has been elicited by the music therapist in a verbal 'guided imagery'. The context may be a walk in the country, a tree or a flower, a gift that one is unwrapping, and so on. The music is not listened to for its own sake, so much as for its potential to evoke and amplify feelings in the client to do with the images evoked.

Here we could say that the music's meaning is strongly referential, in the sense that it is the person's visual/verbal image that is the primary focus of meaning. The music itself is secondary: its role is to enhance the person's pre-existing image. However, there is also an expressionist/absolutist flavour, since the pieces of music are selected very specifically in order to enhance clients' experiences. The music has its own, intrinsic meaning, and is chosen because of its potential to evoke certain feelings in the listener.

Creating Meaning

When Mary Priestley (1988) invites the client to 'play her father' in her improvisation, there is a highly referential component. Here the music is not being improvised so much for its own sake, but rather as representing something other, i.e., how the client feels about her father. Here meaning may be thought of as 'pre-referential' in the sense that the meaning of the music is set *before* the music is created. This is different to referential meaning being assigned or tagged on to music, *after* listening to, or explaining, the event.

In addition, referential meaning is elicited in music therapy when either a client or therapist describes a piece of music as reminding them of something outside the music. In contrast to Guided Imagery in Music, the music may remind them of music that they improvised together in an earlier session (and this they may have assigned certain meaning); it may remind them of something that the therapist and client discussed previously; or the client may make a connection between the music just played and something in his or her life. Here again we need to bear in mind that it is something about the music's form or texture that makes the connection for the person. It is the music itself that evokes the non-musical image.

Therapeutic meaning

It seems however, that music therapists listen 'therapeutically'. Not quite to music as music, nor to structure as structure, but to the person portrayed in the spontaneous music-making. The meaning that they assign to the music will be a therapeutic one, but this will have essences of the various aspects of meaning just described. Let us reconsider the example with Noel.

In the improvisation with Noel, he and I were not merely listening to the music 'out there', as something separate from ourselves, but we were, *together*, part of the music being made. How is meaning generated in such an act: can we 'mean' and create at the same time? Which comes first, the meaning or the creating? Are they distinctive acts, or is the act of creating, itself the meaning? How does the meaning generated during the act of playing colour the meaning in our listening while we play? Are they separate meanings? Do we create the music *in order to* embody a certain meaning that we want to express and convey to the other person? Can our listening be *pure*, in the sense that we are here and the music is there and we do not 'get in the way' of hearing it?

In listening to Noel, I heard *him* in the music: in fact I heard both him and I. I was not listening to his musicianship or to his perceptual prowess. I heard a tightness, busy-ness, rigidity, that told me something about him – in relation to me. (When he showed me his paintings, I recognised the same tightness and busy-ness in his art.) But this is not all I heard.

When Leonard Meyer (1956) speaks of an 'unthinking stimulus', this describes my semi-hypnotised state when improvising with Noel's unchanging and monotonous music. I was on automatic pilot, not at my best therapeutic mode; I had come to expect that the stimulus would remain the same and was, therefore, unstimulated and 'habitual'. When Noel changed what he did, there was a 'block' of my expectant habits: I could no longer be in mesmerised, expectant mode. As Meyer says, it was the change of my expectations that resulted in a heightened state of arousal, switching from an automatic pilot state to one of alertness. Meyer calls this switch an emotional state (and I certainly felt pleasure at the same time). Was it the interruption of the habitual stimulus that was pleasurable in itself? And is this description, drawing loosely from information theory, adequate?

My feeling of excitement at Noel's changes had to do with more than the changes in musical stimulus. As a music therapist, I know that change, especially in the context of being preceded by rigidity, indicates that the potential for extending towards a more fluid 'way of being' is beginning to be realised through music, i.e., the change in Noel's playing could signal the beginning of a more mutual interplay between us, and this, in turn, might signal the beginning of a shift in his own life. These concepts are based on music therapy theory, and they help us to understand, and to explain, what was going on with Noel in the session. Although these theoretical concepts refer to the musical event, they are not musical concepts – they are music therapy concepts. At the moment of change, it was this, together with the 'purely musical' stimulus, that gave me pleasure and excited me. In this sense, my feeling was also referential: it derived from meaning that was not directly musical.

However, this level alone does not constitute music therapy improvisation – and, indeed, we could say that it is the 'other', non-musical level of listening that distinguishes *music* improvisation from *music therapy* improvisation. As music therapists, we create, listen and respond to the improvisation on a non-musical – or an extra-musical – level. This non-musical level is not necessarily referential in the sense of our earlier discussion on absolute and referential meaning.

It seems, then, that there is another level of meaning in music therapy that falls outside this discussion on referential and absolutist meaning in music, and yet is not altogether separate from it. It seems self-evident that music therapists are doing more than just 'playing music' with clients when they improvise together in music therapy sessions, even when they are not assigning referential meaning to the music in the sense described above.

The extra-musical meaning that the therapist 'reads' in the spontaneous, jointly created music improvisation with the client is an interpersonal one. In other words, the therapist is alert to what the music may mean in terms of the interaction between therapist and client, and in terms of the communication between therapist and client. Gary Ansdell (1995) has explained that what matters in clinical improvisation is what is happening in the music *between* the therapist and client, as the music is being created, as the two players share meaning and create a shared meaning through the sounds that they organise between themselves. The music is being read as something 'other' than itself – we can call this the 'clinical-interactive' meaning, and we can see that aspects of both the absolutist and the referentialist positions feature here. This is because it is what goes on *within* the music itself – the way that rhythm, phrasing, intensity or colour develops or fails to develop, that provides cues to the players as to what is going on *between* them. Thus sudden changes, unexpected musical directions, delays in the musical play – all or any of these alert the players, or, to use Meyer's language, heighten their state of arousal. But the meaning does not stop here. The meaning that is assigned to 'what is going on' is not musical meaning – but it is not quite referential meaning either. It is not a meaning 'out there' that is 'unlike' the musical stimulus. In fact the meaning cannot be separated from the music at all.

It is critical to point out, however, that music therapists do not only find alterations or variations or the unexpected meaningful, as information theory suggests. We would also assign therapeutic significance to the fact that there *was* monotony, that the therapist was not paying attention, that there was a lack of variation in what the person was doing in the session. All of these tell us something about the nature of the interaction between therapist and client.

Finally we can see that although music therapy does not quite fit comfortably within any of these theoretical positions, there are some links and overlaps. The absolutist position in music therapy would be a belief that the healing properties lie within the music itself – and perhaps this is derived from the Ancient Greek view that, for example, the Phrygian mode inspires enthusiasm or the Dorian mode produces a relaxed and settled temper (Grout 1960). There was an element of this in my improvisation with Noel: the variation in musical form was significant *in itself.* However, the 'musical' significance is not enough. And, indeed, the musical events may relate directly to aspects of the client's life – which we might call a referentialist position.

More relevant for music therapists, perhaps, is not to polarise absolutism and referentialism, not to think of them as mutually exclusive, and not to ignore that which does not fit neatly into either camp. It might be more useful to consider the various meanings in music as complementing one another, and as enriching our understanding of why and how human beings find music meaningful and intensely significant. This is, after all, one of the tenets underpinning clinical practice. What is becoming clear is that musical meaning is not limited to verbal meaning, and is incomplete and multi-faceted. I want now to look more closely at the signifying function of music, in order to explore, from a slightly different position, the relationship between music and human feeling, and between the personal and the cultural.

Icon, Index and Symbol: A View from Musical Semiotics

The nature of signs

Semiotics is the study of signs: how objects come to have meaning that is generally agreed upon within a culture. For example, how does the word 'cat' come to signal that particular animal within English-speaking culture? The word itself does not look or sound like a cat, neither does it intrinsically portray the qualities of the animal. And yet when we think of the word, we have a sense of that animal's litheness, graceful quickness and alertness. Moreover, the connection between the word 'cat' and the animal is a stable one, developed over hundreds of years, and this enables shared language to become stable. The sign, here, is language: i.e., the word 'cat'. However, the sign could also be a visual representation such as a drawing, or it might be represented by a stone, as part of a children's game. The function of signs is to represent that which is absent. When we use the words 'music therapy' the words are fixed signs, and these have remained sufficiently stable within global culture to enable us to understand (more or less) what the signs refer to, what they mean. The signs are a point of reference. In terms of music, we have seen that music is not simply music – it may present and represent something 'more than' and 'other than' itself. Thinking of music as a sign is immensely complicated, and music therapy, which uses music for a purpose other than itself, necessitates entry into the domain of considering what it is – or how it is – that music signifies.

In thinking about the general characteristics of signs we might ponder on Nattiez' (1990) outline of the characteristics of 'symbolic form'. Nattiez reminds us that the symbol refers. He suggests that the symbolic function is, '…to represent that which is absent' (p.35). By 'referring to' the object, the sign is distanced from the reality of what it refers to, and the space that is created between the sign and its object is a social and a cultural one – although in music therapy I would suggest that the space between the sign (music) and its object may also be very personal and idiosyncratic. The general function of signs is to mediate between 'the discourse' (or the musical text) and what the discourse represents. The sign is autonomous in the sense of having its own domain and of being explicable on its own terms. A sign, also, is a thing: it evolves and effects, it modifies and influences its environment. The symbolic exists: it is real rather than a private mental construct. Nattiez suggests that the use of the term 'symbolic form' refers to music's capacity to, 'give rise to a complex and infinite web of interpretants' (p.37).

In terms of the signalling function of music, semioticians refer to the work of Charles Pierce (1932), who suggested that messages of all kinds are a function of three interactants: an object (the music), an interpretant (the 'agent' who does the signifying or makes the link – although, as Nattiez reminds us, this link may already be culturally established), and a sign (that is, the emotion, which is used to signify). Pierce described the classification of signs into the three categories of index, icon or symbol, as the most fundamental division of signs. It is the manner in which the sign relates to the object, rather than the object itself, that distinguishes between icon, index and symbol. These distinctions provide a useful, if highly theoretical and general, starting point in thinking of the signifying function of music (Figure 2.2).

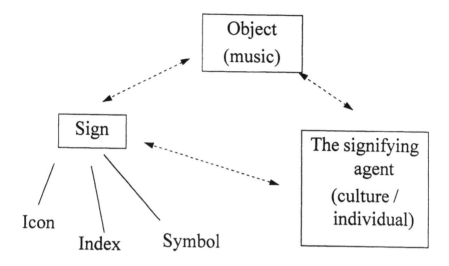

Figure 2.2 The relationship between the object, its sign and the signifying agent

MUSIC AS SYMBOL

We may, for example, think of music as being *symbolic*. Here, like the referentialists, we are linking one thing (the music) to another (the symbol), but the link between the two is an arbitrary one in the sense that the symbol does not especially resemble its object (or the word 'cat' does not look or sound like the animal). Once the link between a thing and its object is made, the continuous association between that particular music and that particular symbol remains fixed. However, symbols can grow and become transformed by human beings drawing from old symbols to create new ones. For our purposes, this means that the association between the music and the symbol is not a spontaneous one that differs at different hearings of the same piece of music.

For example, a piece of music may be identified by a society as symbolising something for that society. Thus an anthem such as 'N'khosi Sikhelele Afrika' has enormously powerful emotional resonances, initially as symbolising the struggle against apartheid in South Africa and, more recently, as a symbol of that country's new beginning. We call its meaning symbolic because, like all symbols, there is nothing inherent in that music – in its melody or harmonic texture – that tells us of a struggle and victory against a repressive regime. Rather, through its use by people within a culture over a particular period of social upheaval, it has acquired meaning which is difficult, if not impossible, to disassociate from the music itself. We could say that it is through being associated with the anti-apartheid struggle over a long period of time, that this anthem now has particular emotional significance for people of that culture. The association is fixed in the sense that it is very difficult to hear this anthem without its symbolic association and, at the same time, the quality of this association has become transformed over the years, as the culture of 'struggle' has given way to a 'struggling democracy'.

MUSIC AS ICON

Another way of considering the meaningfulness of music is the *iconic* view: an icon is linked to that which it represents by resembling it or by capturing a quality of that object. A drawing of a cat is iconic, in that we can see immediately by looking at the drawing what it represents. In terms of music, we could say that music holds meaning for us because something about it resembles human emotion: the ebb and flow, tensions and relaxations in music resemble the ebb and flow, tension and relaxation of human feeling. There are two trends of thought supporting this view, one being that of Suzanne Langer (1951), who supports earlier views held by Eduard Hanslick, that music represents non-specific emotions. Langer suggests that music reflects what she calls a 'morphology of feelings' – i.e., it reflects their patterns of tension and resolution, the dynamic shifts of human emotions. Emotions are formalised and articulated in what she calls 'significant form' – music portrays not anger, joy, excitement, but rather, the *properties* of these feelings.

MUSIC AS INDEX

However, another way of thinking about the meaning of music is that music, quite simply, affects us directly, rather than affecting us *because* it is associated with something else or because we recognise an aspect of ourselves within the music. This direct effect of music is the *indexical* view, and here music simply has direct access to and from our emotional life. We are directly affected by it: the index is connected with its object, the two can be seen as an 'organic pair', and their relationship is a natural, rather than a cultivated, one.

Comments on Music as Sign: Music and Music Therapy

All of these concepts acknowledge that music – all music, not just in music therapy – has a relationship with human emotion in the broadest sense of the word. Music and emotion have 'something in common', based on a similarity between the two or, as Langer puts it, music reflects the morphology (i.e. the shape or texture) of feelings. Humans recognise patterns of flow, fluctuation or dissolution, of sustained or sudden tension and resolution, manifested in music. Moreover we are affected by these patterns: there exists an inextricable link between these patterns and human response to them, although this link is not a fixed one. Rather we are susceptible to music because its forms already exist in our minds.

As with the absolutist and referentialist debate, we need to be careful about thinking in terms of mutually exclusive positions, i.e. that meaning is either indexical, symbolic or iconic. Rather, we can think that what makes us read symbolic meaning into a musical event is because the music has a direct emotional effect on us (indexical), and this effect helps to forge the link between the music and its symbolic representation and significance. Moreover, something in the form of the music may indeed resemble (iconic) an aspect of what the music comes to symbolise. Thus the symbol may well have some iconic qualities: we might say, for example, that there is something about the morphology of 'N'khosi Sikhelele Afrika' that renders it a particularly potent symbol. For me its morphology is sluggish and dragging, which symbolises the sagging spirits of African people in the 'struggle' years in South Africa. The indexical view, that suggests that music affects or stimulates our psyche directly because something of its quality is already encoded in our minds, can be represented here because my mind already 'knows' what 'sagging, dragging' is/looks like/sounds like, and my mind is receptive to being stimulated by the 'sagging and dragging' in the music. The relationship between music and mind will be explored through a different discourse later in this book.

In contrast to the significance of 'Nkhosi Sikhelele Afrika', which has a substantial public and cultural significance, in music therapy we can think of the therapist and client negotiating meaning and significance between them. Here we see that music therapists employ all three of Pierce's categories of signs, depending on their theoretical orientation. Some may make verbal interpretations on the improvised music because of its iconic character, checking with patients (or inviting them to check) whether the music sounds sad or angry, because its texture and shape reminds them of the texture and shape of angry feelings, or of excited feelings, and so on. Thus I recognised the texture of tightness in Noel's playing as signifying something outside the music; signifying something about him – and about us. This recognition was iconic. At other times therapists may work in the symbolic mode, and encourage patients to make the association between, for example, a slow improvised tango and its symbolic representation of passion and romance.

(What, then, was the symbolism of our improvisation for Noel?) Patients may also volunteer their own associations: a link that has been formed for them between the music and something that happened in their lives. Here the symbolism is personal, rather than cultural, as in the tango music.

We also see that the indexical, or the direct, relationship between the music and the therapist and client enables the formation of an authentic, if transitory, emotional bond between the patient and therapist. Perhaps it is this indexical relationship that embodies the true function of music, at the root of the power that music has over us. Karbusicky (1987), in particular, puts forward a strong case for the immediacy of the effect of music. It is this immediacy which can be elicited by using musical improvisation in a particular way in music therapy. Thus we could say that Noel 'needed' to play his tightness, by 'reversing' the indexical relationship. In other words, his personal tightness has a direct effect on the music that he spontaneously played. At the same time, however, he – or rather, we – were directly affected by it: both of us felt his tightness, presented in sound. The music affected us directly, bypassing symbolic meaning and, to some extent, iconic significa-tion, and was the bond between us at the moment.

In Theory and Practice

We saw in the first chapter that the relationship between theory and practice is complex and multi-faceted. What has become increasingly clear in this discussion is that the theory of semiotics helps music therapists to frame music improvisation within the context of a distinctive theoretical discourse that examines the meaning of the musical act in human life.

In thinking about semiotics, we see that the music therapist herself has access to a system of signs that we might label 'music therapy theory'. This discourse is language-based, although it is often inspired by non-linguistic events, and, like language, it has evolved over years of professional develop-ment, of thinking about the work, of writing and reading about it. Within this discourse, certain improvisational events are assigned special signifi-cance, and when these occur (as with, for example, Noel changing his playing), the 'green light' goes on inside the therapist's mind (with Noel, I became excited, my level of anticipation rose). Here we might say that the therapist taps into theory in order to make sense of what is going on in the practice. At the same time, however, we see that the therapist is directly affected by the music (the indexical view) and, in addition, we might use Leonard Meyer's information theory to explain how the inhibition of expectation in the therapist gave rise to her feeling of excitement.

The therapist's private meaning – which may make use of various theoretical discourses as well as her personal experience – then needs to be 'negotiated' with the client's own private meaning, which is unlikely to be based on music therapy theory, but on his personal life. In this way, a shared and mutual meaning may begin to emerge out of the session. With Noel, we spoke about what happened, after playing, and reached a mutual point of acknowledging the significance of what had happened.

But what if Noel were physically disabled? What if his body did not do what he wanted to express: what would happen to the morphology of feelings? What would happen to the iconic signification, and how would that affect the symbolic and the indexical effect? How would we review, and renew, how 'whisperings and stormings' sound?

And, further, what if Noel were 'mad', and the meaning of the event so distorted that I could not rely on culturally generated signification to share with him the 'sense' and 'meaning' of what occurred? If Noel were 'mad', how would we enter his private 'discourse of madness'?

Unsurprisingly, given that she was a philosopher primarily concerned with aesthetics, Suzanne Langer's view that music reflects the morphology of feelings stops short of what we might call 'feelings distorted by mental illness', and does not begin to address the 'crisis of meaning' that accompanies mental disturbance (McNamee 1992). At the beginning of this chapter, Nattiez reminded us that music consists of various dimensions, including the process of creating music and the process of receiving it and reconstructing it in our minds, as well as the analysing of it, of its structure and forms. Each of these acts 'means' differently, and none of them in isolation consists of music. To this, music therapists might add dimensions of complexity, to do with the interpersonal nature of the musical act and to do with the meaning of, and meaning in, the client's pathology.

In music therapy we have seen that meaning is not just to do with the relationship between the music improvisation as object and the significance of its referent. Meaning, in music therapy, is also to do with what happens between therapist and client. Meaning has many facets, and in the next chapter this exploration into meaning is extended towards music as a universal, and a culture-specific, phenomenon.

CHAPTER 3

Music Therapy and Universals
Between Culture and Compromise

This chapter explores the meaning of music therapy as a universal *and* as a culture-specific phenomenon, in an attempt at addressing a basic premise in support of music therapy: that humans are susceptible to the power of music since it is a universal phenomenon and since it exists in all human beings.

The phenomenon of music is universal in the sense that music exists in all cultures. Moreover, some would say that all world musics have features in common that transcend culture specificity: at the very least, all world musics have beat, melody and most use instruments that are beaten, plucked, strummed, blowed or bowed. How useful is the concept of music universals for music therapists? At the other end of the spectrum, how useful is the idea of culture specificity? In this chapter I move between these two positions, and explore the use of cross-cultural music in music therapy practice and music therapy in cross-cultural contexts, as well as examining music universals from the perspective of music therapy. First, the discipline is contextualised within cultural concepts of music/illness/health/healing, and the theoretical discourse here is that of ethnomusicology and social psychology.

The Universality of Music

The concept of the 'universality' of music is usually understood as meaning that music has existed in all human cultures and continues to do so, whether the cultures are remote, rural or tribal, or whether they are urban, industrial, post-industrial and technologically 'plugged in'. What constitutes a 'culture' needs some attention, especially with the transient nature of many cultures today. Some cultures are stable: for example, people from a social class, people who have lived in the same area for generations and people who, for generations, have subscribed to, and been part of, particular religious rituals. Some cultures are temporary: migrant labourers in many countries alternate between rural and urban lifestyles and even between one country and another; there are people who live in an area at a certain time and then move on (to retire, for instance), people who support a political cause at a certain time of their lives, people of a particular age group who frequent clubs that play certain kinds of music, or, for that matter, music therapists who have trained in a specific method, who practise with a particular client group, who are enthusiastic about research or who are burnt-out.

Each of these cultures and subcultures has defining features, which may be ideological, may be identified by a particular way of dressing or by attending culture-specific rituals, and so on. Each of these cultures and subcultures can also be seen as identifying with a particular kind of music, which they listen to, dance to and play. In some instances, we could say that a particular music typifies or defines a group or subculture, and is a powerful uniting influence. Moreover, a specific music may well be identified globally as belonging to that culture. For example, we identify the reggae music of Bob Marley with Rastafarian culture, flamenco music with Spanish gypsy culture and Gospel music with Christian worship in parts of North America.

Many of us who live in technologised societies have the extraordinary freedom to choose, to some extent, which musical culture we wish to enter. We may tap into Northern Indian classical music, French Renaissance dance music or the epic ballads of Aberzadjan, for example, and each of these gives us a sense, a taste, an impression of other people and other places, and other concepts of time. To hear any of these on a CD player is rather a different experience to 'being there', in which case we can also imbibe the colours, smells and social context of the music. All of these are part of the music experience.

For example, I once heard a group of Mozambican drummers playing in downtown Johannesburg, and was drawn to the piazza where this was happening. What soon became evident was the cultural differences between people's experience of the music. The Africans seemed to go on their daily business, hawking, talking, walking past, almost as though the music were not occurring. Some occasionally joined the drummers and the dancers for a short burst and would then leave and continue on their daily business. In contrast, the non-Africans sat and listened to the music, mostly in silence, as though it were a concert performance. For some people, music was part of the day and you simply went about your business, whereas for others it was a seperate event. This ambience, of course, coloured my experience of the music itself in a way very different to my listening to a CD of this drumming in a CD store in London's Oxford Street.

This example draws attention to the very different functions and roles of music in different societies. Martin Stokes (1994) reports that for the Suya people of Brazil, music and dance performance helps to articulate social time, the cosmology and social organisation, whereas the rural migrant workers of Chile identify with urban musical genres in order to transform themselves into urbanites while they are in the city. Both of these experiences are different to our own technologised and industrialised existence, where rituals (whether accompanied by music or not) have become peripheral, and the music that we listen to (in contrast to the music that we are forced to hear, daily) is slotted into gaps created by the working day and the working week. In downtown Johannesburg, some of us stopped what we were doing in order to listen, whereas others apparently listened while going about their daily business.

Stokes suggests that listening to music can also *transform* our social space. If we think of music as being socially meaningful in this way, we can see that it helps us to create a space within which we recognise, and identify with, our culture, as well as the boundaries that separate our culture from others. For example, the 12-year-old in our household, while happy to sing along to music by the Beatles, Joan Baez, Sting or Nina Simone, also defines 'her' music, which we are not invited to share or even to listen to. Some of the music belongs to the 'family' culture, and some to her own and that of her peers. At a conference I once had an experience of an exclusive and unexpected cultural space being created, spontaneously, through culture-specific music, despite understanding the words and the musical structure. There were many conference social gatherings, some organised and others spontaneous, after each day's papers and workshops. During one of the evening social gatherings, various participants had put together a variety concert, part of which consisted of a woman leading the audience in various songs. Since I knew most of the songs, or at least the tunes, I joined in the singing and felt part of the general bonhomie of a large body of people singing together. Then she began a song which was totally unfamiliar to me, despite having lived in Britain for many years. I recall clearly the instant feeling of exclusion, and looked around to see whether I was alone. After this event, in speaking to others who were also not singing, we discussed our feelings, which were aggravated by the fact that everyone else seemed to know the song, the words, and, more frustrating still, there seemed to be inferences to the song that people seemed to know and were laughing about. Until this song was sung, we had all felt part of the group, part of the shared affective experience and part of the 'conference culture' that had been embodied by the singing. The song created an instant, though temporary, boundary between those of us who were foreign – despite being English-speaking – and those who were part of British culture.

Despite the presence of musical universals, we know that the music of other cultures is by no means directly accessible – even if we understand the words of, say, a particular song. Hidden nuances and symbolism are subtly, and exclusively, cultural. Dowling and Harwood (1986) suggest that much of our knowledge about the music of our own culture is tacit and implicit, unbound by explicit verbalisation or textbooks. They give a delightful description of Dane Harwood's attempts, over several years, to strike the *gong ageng* of the Gamelan set at the right time and with the right sound: there seemed to be no appropriate description of what was correct, apart from direct observation and the smiles of the Javanese musicians with whom he played.

Music therapists who develop improvisation techniques as part of their training are encouraged to familiarise themselves with the music of different cultures. This is not so much in order to distinguish between clients belonging to a particular culture, but rather to familiarise ourselves with the differences in 'musical energy' that different world musics may embody. This energy is culture-specific in the sense that it may be portrayed by particular musical styles and idioms. Music therapists might draw from a particular musical genre in an improvisation, as reflecting and evoking something within the client's playing. (Here we are taken back to the iconic sign, in the sense that a musical genre might *resemble* something that the music therapist recognises in the client's playing.) Also, the therapist, in an improvisation, might choose to introduce a certain music in order to elicit or trigger a quality that she senses is latent in the client's playing.

Despite being confined by the use of tempered tuning of Western musical instruments, music therapists might explore, for example, the Spanish idiom, which has rather a different texture and impulse to, say, the highly defined harmonic and rhythmic structure of the blues, boogie woogie or the tango of Buenos Aires. Nordoff and Robbins (1971) suggest that there are inherent therapeutic qualities that are generated by the distinctive emotional–tonal– melodic characteristic of different world musics, such as Balinese, Slavonic, Latin American, Scottish, Arabian, Oriental and other ethnic musics. They approach this from the concept of archetypes in music, that enable us to tap into music that transcends our own culture and geography, because of the inherent qualities of these genres. Different musics have, undoubtedly, different qualities that affect us directly: most of us cannot listen to sub-Saharan African music without moving our hips to it, whereas a Scottish Peobruch hardly elicits the same response.

For example, I once worked with a rather ebullient Scottish man from a mining community in eastern Scotland. His being thoroughly Scottish in culture might have suggested music in the Scots idiom – but that would have been rather facile and may have been counter-empathic. In our work together it was the Latin American tango that first checked his rather loud, repetitive, almost militaristic beating on the snare drum. The tango, on the conga drum, seemed to crystallise his virile machismo and his prodigious vitality (which often found expression in aggressive acts), as well as evoking a deep-seated sensitivity and gracefulness which I intuited both clinically and musically. This was quite apart from the rhythmic pattern of the tango which 'caught' him. The tango, as we used it, evoked a latent spaciousness within him, so that after this we quickly moved towards exquisitely graceful waltzes with rubatos that would have done Chopin proud. As we shall see later, the critical feature of our improvisations was not that the man had to perfect the use of that Latin American idiom, but rather that he was able to tap into its musical energy and quality, and this propelled him towards a broader, more complex, experience of himself.

In one sense, then, to think of using other 'world musics' is, in fact, to use them in a way that is limited by our own cultural conventions, and by our limited grasp of their significance. We can only use other world musics within our own comfort and effectiveness. Despite these limitations, defined by our own culturally bound experience of music, the music of other cultures is, in some instances, sufficiently translatable into our own for us to gain something from it.

Movement patterns

John Baily (1985) draws our attention to another phenomenon which is as much culture-bound as it is universal: the idea that musical patterns are not only mental representations, but are patterns of movement in relation to the shape of the musical instrument that the music is played on. For example, he discusses at length the spatial properties of the Afghan rubab and the Herati dutar, which are culture-specific, in relation to the human sensorimotor system. The combination of these influences the shape of the music, and Baily suggests that African music may be thought of as movement representation rather than an auditory one.

The fact that the patient described earlier played on an untuned percussion instrument at the time of the tango, was a specific sensorimotor experience which undoubtedly influenced his emotional experience of the music. Playing a conga drum (usually played standing up) emphasises rather narrow, vertical movements, which would lend greater weight to the accents when he needed them. The Chopinesque waltz was played on the metallophone, and this is a different spatial experience, with the combination of vertical and horizontal movements, as well as the very different timbre of the instruments. The metallophone, of course, resonates for longer than the conga drum, and this may have encouraged a lilt in his playing that was not evident in earlier, tight beating on the snare drum.

Leslie Bunt (1994) takes great care in writing about the different timbres of instruments used in music therapy, while Nordoff and Robbins (1971) emphasise the direct, active engagement of a child beating a drum in music therapy. The movement activates the child's emotional life. They write: 'The music is in movement – the child's emotional experiences are also in movement...the vital life of feeling becomes united with perceiving, with intelligent comprehension and with action – and all are integrated by the essential individuality of the child in communicative expressiveness' (pp.50, 51).

Gary Ansdell alerts us to the quality of movement of an animate body: in contrast to a machine, an animate body has flow, continuity, co-ordination, purpose and direction – and we know from the work of Bengtsson (1980) and of Gabrielsson (1982) that where highly sophisticated synthesisers may be able to reproduce all of these in sound, what they lack is the essential micro-mis-timings that lend an essential 'human-ness' to movement – what Bengtsson and Gabrielsson call 'systematic variations' in rhythmical performance.

Universal structural bases

John Sloboda (1985) cautiously suggests that despite the absence of cognitive modelling of non-Western music, there exist within the amazing musical diversity of musical cultures across the globe, recognisable structural bases. At the very least, these universals render certain aspects of music that sounds very 'alien' accessible to us. In his comparison of sub-Saharan and North African music, he alerts us to the rhythmic strength and vitality, the polyphonic, the call–response form of sub-Saharan music in contrast to the monophonic, solo, vocal emphasis of North African music. All of these qualities are accessible to Western musicians because they fall within our realm of musical experience: we can imagine solo versus group music, the call–answer format, the voice versus the emphasis on beating, rhythmic vitality, and so on – although we undoubtedly imagine them from within our cultural moulds. Music 'universals' correspond to how we perceive musical structure (which is addressed later in this book). What is interesting, from a music therapy point of view, is that some of these music universals are central to music therapists' clinical interest, not so much from a neurological or perceptual – or cultural – position, but rather, from an inter-personal one, as we shall see later.

Universality in Music

A discussion on features that are found in musics of various cultures cannot be separated from exploring how human beings perceive music 'in their minds', so to speak. We know that our minds favour patterning: we seek patterns in order to make sense of our environment, and where there are apparently none (e.g. in the starlit sky), we impose them in a way that fits most comfortably with our mental structures. In creating music – especially with other people – we need to ensure that its patterns are accessible to them as well as to ourselves: we need to share patterning.

John Blacking (1987) suggests that the mind in a 'natural' state, unfettered by social and cultural conventions, reveals what he terms 'cognitive universals', that all human beings share. Thus music that is based on universal mental structures will resonate with listeners who are unfamiliar with the cultural idiom. Here universality is in the human mind, and is reflected in the music that is created by human minds. But is this view sufficient? I have had direct experience of playing apparently simple African rhythms and feeling 'out of step' and unable to enter into the complexity of even a regular beat – which is, after all, a biological universal (Pavlicevic 1996a). The discussion below is drawn from Sloboda (1985), Dowling and Harwood, (1986) and Howell, Cross and West (1985).

One of the universal features of music all over the world is that music takes place within fixed reference pitches. These pitches are selected from a large set of tonal material, and once a piece of music begins, the discrete pitches that have been selected as part of that piece remain constant for the duration of the piece of music being performed. (Think of the Indian classical musician who defines the raga before beginning it – thereby establishing a tonal framework for the listener). Moreover, the principal reference pitch is often sustained throughout the piece in the form of a drone, and this provides a perceptual anchor for that piece of music. Within many cultures, some pitches appear more frequently, and the piece of music moves around them or refers to them in such a way as to leave the listener with little doubt as to its privilege.

If we look at the concept of the scale system across cultures, it appears that within most scales the octave is a particularly privileged interval, often reinforcing the principal reference pitch with doubling or trebling. In most cultures, the notion of a scale and a tonic have formal analogies with tonality, whether the scale is tonal or not, and the subdivision of the octave into scale steps is found in most cultures, with five- and seven-note scales being particularly common. In no culture is the division of the scale within the octave into equal ratios, and the uneven intervals help us to get our musical bearings: points of more or less tension orientate us towards potential resolution around the tonic note of the scale.

If we now turn our attention to the universal significance of timing (which is, after all, such a fundamental aspect of our humanity, both biologically, mentally and spiritually), we see that 'reference times' provide a focus in relation to which other sounds are organised. In many cultures instruments are used to mark out a regular pulse or metre. These fixed points of rhythm and of melody provide musicians with cues of synchrony, enabling them to anticipate and adjust their musical behaviour so as to co-ordinate with what the other players are doing. Ethnomusicologist John Blacking (1973) has shown that in sub-Saharan music, which is predominantly social in nature in the sense that music is part of social rituals or, indeed, of any gathering, the prominence of the beat has a unifying effect for the group. We could say that most dance musics of the world emphasise the beat, which enables people to hear the music 'in the same way', and move with it together – in a way that they could not move to, say, Debussy's 'La Mer'.

Negotiating Culture in Music Therapy

In music therapy improvisation, we can think in terms of the therapist and client together negotiating their own musical culture, and one of the basic clinical features of playing together is that of jointly defining and establishing a mutually comfortable beat. This means that the beat is not imposed by either one or the other player, but is negotiated mutually by both players. Indeed the shared beat is given prominence in clinical work, as signifying the establishment of a relationship through music improvisation. The joint beat can be seen as a shared universal, underpinning and enabling both players to share the music, so to speak, to create music jointly (much as improvising musicians do) rather than tugging against one another in order to maintain their individual beat.

Leslie Bunt (1994) draws our attention to the musical behaviour of people – adults and children – with profound learning difficulties. He describes a lack of understanding that one pulse can precede and generate another: Bunt calls this a form of pre-pulse behaviour. The musical acts that he describes have a lack of shape, an absence of predictability and show a randomness of events. This is not unlike my experience of playing with severely depressed patients, where the absence of volition and the flattening of motor activity result in long, unpredictable gaps that are very difficult for the music therapist to meet. Music therapists need to be able to anticipate clients' playing. Nordoff and Robbins again:

> If a child shows in his beating a limited rhythmic awareness or a lack of rhythmical continuity, your main goal will almost always be to lead him into beating and experiencing the basic beat. Very often, on this level, you will be working to establish contact with a child who is communicatively isolated. (1971, p.135)

In terms of the universality of a time referent, both as a social phenomenon and as a reflection of our neurological cohesiveness, music therapists know that one of the musical manifestations of communication deficits in patients is the incapacity to establish and sustain the 'basic beat' – or the musical pulse. This is an interesting metaphor, in that we could see it as imaging these patients' remaining at the periphery of their culture, without access to the 'essential' aspect of belonging to humanity, i.e. that of sharing and exchanging meaning through human communication. For example, as part of a research study on music therapy and the rehabilitation of persons suffering from chronic schizophrenia (Pavlicevic, Trevarthen and Duncan 1994), I began to understand the musical manifestation of communication deficits in schizophrenia, through the absence of a mutually established, reciprocal use of the beat. We know that a psychological aspect of the illness is an incapacity to establish and sustain relationships with the 'outside' world: the schizophrenic person has no clear sense of boundary, i.e. what belongs to the outside world and what is part of the inner world. This incapacity is manifested musically in several ways, all of which centre around the difficulty in establishing a beat that is shareable.

For example, an elderly man whom I shall call Frank, had the most rigid and inflexible beat imaginable. In terms of establishing a relationship with him, I did all the 'meeting'. For as long as I played on his beat we were 'together', although in a rather stilted and one-sided way. His playing could not accommodate the slightest change, and any variation on my part would result in us parting musical company. Here was a truly narrow time referent (in this instance the pulse), which was barely 'musical' in character. In terms of a therapeutic relationship, this was what I came to call one-way contact (Pavlicevic 1995a). Most performing musicians will understand this kind of situation without needing to read it therapeutically. As a flautist, I recall the nightmare of having accompanists who did not move 'with' me: despite the more explicit aspects of the beat being shared, the subtle nuances, in these instances, were not.

With another schizophrenic man, Derek, we were at the other polarity to Frank. Derek's playing was utterly chaotic and disorganised, and there was simply no hint of a musical pulse. I spent a long time floundering in my own playing when attempting to 'find' him. Eventually I realised that I would have to provide a time referent for us both – although this might at first put paid to a musical relationship, since I would be playing in a fixed time rather than attempting to meet his chaos. Gradually I began to discern his emerging attempts at connecting with me. We began to move together rather tenuously, in some kind of common time frame, despite his playing remaining extraordinarily disorganised. However, an accent here or there coincided sufficiently with my steady playing to suggest a loosely defined communication between us.

We might say that in the case of Derek, we both began to move towards creating a musical culture of our own: one that would suit both of us, one which was an expression of the combination of us as human beings. With Frank, in contrast, I remained 'culturally alienated': we were only together when I entered his world – he imposed his world on to me, and I was in the position of being 'colonised', so to speak.

If we think of music from very different geographical cultures, do the universals in music help us in any way to have access to that music? It would seem that where the unfamiliar music can more or less fit into our own mental framework, we are able to make sense of some of it.

For example, I once worked with a group of women in Johannesburg as part of a short programme on music-as-communication with handicapped persons. I asked them to sing a song that they knew, so that we could together look at its potential for developing appropriate movements with their clients. After some discussion in their vernacular, they sang a rural Tswana rain song, of which I understood not a word. However, after one hearing I had a fairly clear sense of the overall structure (which was by no means clear-cut), which I checked out with them by describing the song as something like this. First you did a fast bit and you did that a second time (AA). Then there was another bit that had less rhythm (B), and then there was another bit that was different from that bit (C). Then you did the first, fast bit again, but only once (A), and then you did the second other bit that had less rhythm (B), and then again the fast bit from the beginning, once (A). Then you did something different (D), and the quiet bit again (B) and then the fast bit again (A). In my mind the sequence went something like: A–A–B–C–A–B–A–D–B–A.

It did not matter that the contents of each section were a closed book in terms of the cultural and symbolic associations of the song, or that I could not quite reconcile the pentatonic-like tune with its diatonic harmonising.

The musical cues that I needed were in the form of pitch and time referents, which are trans-culturally accessible. The accents alerted me to the metre or a cross-rhythm, a change of pace defined the pace preceding it, a particular rhythm repeated at certain points defined a preceding section, and in-between bits, although different from one another, had similar lengths, so that I could identify the various sections.

Despite the gap between our cultures, there was enough that was familiar to me in the structure of the song – and here it must be borne in mind that much African traditional music has become hybridised: the result of zealous Christian missionaries who quickly saw that the 'infidel' could be reached through traditional hymns. The group and I were quickly able to reach a common understanding about what we could do with this particular song, so that we could begin to work with it.

However, there was another dimension that highlighted the difference between our cultures, and which supports Dane Harwood's difficulty with his Gamelan playing. Since most African cultures do not separate music from movement, part of my assimilating the song's structure was to dance with the women while they were singing it. The steps were not especially complicated, but I was aware of lacking the culture-bound nuances of dancing. My distinctly 'European' rendering of the movements, although accurate in time and in terms of the steps themselves, lacked the wiggle here, the sigh there, the heavy woosh that made the movements singularly African. As Dane Harwood explains, there are subtleties that are highly culture-specific and that are inaccessible to outsiders – thus even if we do use the idioms of other cultures in music therapy improvisation, we do so within a highly localised context that can only reproduce an aspect of that culture's music.

Do we talk about cross-cultural music therapy? Do those of us who work with people from cultures that are different to our own think in these terms? I am not aware of using specifically African idioms when working with African people in South Africa, even in work with people who do not share the same verbal language. However, in my group work with children from Johannesburg townships, I cannot separate music from movement: a significant component of the sessions is, in fact, to do with movement – and I suppose that this is a cross-cultural phenomenon (Pavlicevic 1994). My feeling is that there is an implicit degree of inculturation that has taken place by the time clients from another culture find themselves in music therapy. This implies an acknowledgement of the presence of illness or pathology according to Western thinking, and an acknowledgement also of therapy being something to do with healing. Despite a poor command of English, the children at one Johannesburg school know that they need to 'have problems' in order to come to music therapy. Being African, some of these children's families consult Sangomas, or traditional healers, who have a different, and more complex, understanding of 'illness' and 'problems'. However, the apparent differences in the understanding of 'problems' do not seem to be a difficulty in working with these children.

Culturally Learned Meaning in Music Therapy

The use of pre-composed music in music therapy – especially of traditional or folk music – raises the issue of culture-specificity and culturally bound meaning. Highly defined – and confined – association (i.e., symbolic meaning), is usually culture-specific, and this may well prevent any other level of meaning from emerging in a music therapy session. Where therapist and client share the same culture, the use of a particular musical idiom that has strong connotations can be problematic.

For example, in a music therapy session with a young woman (from a similar cultural background to mine), our joint improvisation seemed to me to be moving rather obviously towards 'What Shall we Do with the Drunken Sailor?' and I arrived at it playing with great gusto, affirmed by the young woman's energetic and exuberant playing. Or so I thought. After the session she told me that she was extremely irritated: she felt offended, the music was trivial, and what did a song such as this have to do with our work? I felt chastised by the vehemence of her telling off, but at the same time shared with her my intuition, which was that I had never before heard her play with so much focus and energy. On reflection, I was left with uncertainty as to whether I had been insensitive because of the wording of that particular song – this was, in a sense, confirmed by her irritation and frustration, clearly linked to the culturally bound meaning of the song. With a song such as this, its associations are so established that anyone from that culture would find it very difficult to hear it 'afresh', so to speak. In our session, this limited the young woman's conscious emotional experience to one of irritation and annoyance with me: her experience was that my use of the song in our session offended her. Moreover, her focusing on the highly definite meaning of the song prevented her from hearing and experiencing something quite different, i.e., her free-flowing energy which was, undoubtedly, fuelled by her annoyance. This was the dimension that I felt was the more significant, therapeutically.

Music Therapy as a Social Event

I want to look briefly at the music therapy event as a 'social' one, drawing parallels with music psychologists (Atik 1995; Davidson 1996) who have looked at music performance as a social phenomenon. Within any culture, there are culture-specific expectations about what music therapy is: in the 'developed' world, music therapy fits more or less into the inherited tradition of the healer/patient dichotomy and of traditional models of illness and the need for treatment.

However, the music therapy event generates its own explicit and negotiated 'rules' that we might think of as the 'etiquette' of therapy: for example, arriving and leaving at a certain time, negotiating arrangements to do with time, length, place of appointment, remuneration of therapist, and so on. (These 'social rules', of course, can also be understood within the psychodynamic discourse of 'therapeutic frames' which we shall explore later.) This etiquette paves the way for the spontaneous event inside the music therapy session. Seen through this 'social psychology' lens, the music therapy session can be seen as one of collaboration between therapist and client, of co-ordination and co-operation – in other words, a mutual willingness to take part in this event.

In terms of the social rules of music therapy, we might think also of the therapist being 'appraised', especially in early sessions, for her skills and her ability to communicate, which contribute to the client appraising the therapist negatively or positively – or a bit of both. I would like to propose that, at the same time, the therapist is, albeit subtly, appraising the client: something along the lines of, 'can I work with this person; is there a "chemistry" between us which will inhibit or aid the work; is this person "suitable" as a client', and so on.

Jane Davidson (1996) draws attention to the 'group function' of successful string quartets; these include members having a 'sense of affiliation' to the group and individuals feeling a common connection between them, as well as a feeling of interdependence, built on trust and respect of individual boundaries. In addition, successful string quartet leaders are flexible, being both directive and democratic. These concepts are 'borrowable' by music therapists. It seems that both client and therapist need a sense of commitment, and of 'belonging' to the therapy sessions. Also, both partners are dependent on one another for the session to happen at all: the session cannot happen if either the client or the therapist does not respect the etiquette negotiated at the start of sessions. We can also think of the music itself transforming the social space created by the negotiated etiquette.

A Final Note

I have always been curious about the existence of discussions about the universality of music, since they invariably treat music as a phenomenon 'out there' to which human beings have some magical link. If we consider the musical ingredients of pulse, pitch, timbre and texture to be part of our neurological and biological functioning, then it seems odd to think in these exteriorised terms.

The following chapters explore in some detail the processes involved in listening to music and in responding to it, in a way that removes us from our musical cultures and focuses on the human experience of sound. What these descriptions make clear is that the *universality in music* as well as the *universality of music* have psychological and neurological substance; this complements the above discussion and lends weight to the statements that music therapists are especially fond of: that we are all 'music beings'. This is because, as we shall see, the universals in music are also 'music universals in humans': music universals are part of our physical and mental life.

CHAPTER 4

With Rigour and Imagination
Music Therapy and Music Psychology

Reading snow is like listening to music.
To describe what you've read is to try to explain music in writing.
(Peter Høeg: *Miss Smilla's Feeling for Snow*)

Facts and Fiction

The delightful Miss Smilla more than manages to convey and to evoke the subtleties and complexities of snow, so that in reading those words, I experienced directly its marvellous bleakness and terrible beauty. Why is it, then, that although music psychologists have put together verbal information about music perception and cognition, much of their writing leaves me with no sense of what music is, beyond words that are dry, flat, horizontal and thoroughly brittle?

There is, of course, a distinction to be made between evocative writings that are works of art and factual or informative writings that convey general information with no attempt to 'colour' facts. However, in thinking about where and how the disciplines of music therapy and music psychology might talk with one another, I have found it useful to think in terms of the 'nomothetic' in contrast to the 'idiographic' approaches to the study of events.

A nomothetic approach is a more general and abstract drawing up of 'rules' that might be said to be true for all people. Here information might be very generalised, and applicable to the general characteristics of, say, snow and ice. This gives us some idea about it, but at the same time this information cannot convey the very different qualities of snow, for example, in Africa on Mount Kilimanjaro, and snow in Scandinavian countries in the white bleakness of the Arctic Circle. An idiographic description, in contrast, offers richly textured details of unique events, not unlike Miss Smilla's exquisite and highly personal account of snow and ice. However, we need to be cautious here: while Miss Smilla's account is highly evocative in the context of her narrative, it may not necessarily offer all that there is to know about icy conditions. Her descriptions are not necessarily appropriate ones on which to base general information of snow and ice, which can be transferred from the Arctic Circle to the African Peaks. We might say that her idiographic descriptions (individualised and detailed) complement more general – i.e., nomothetic – information that we already have about temperature, humidity, climate and geography to offer us a sensuous and chilling experience. Indeed we might argue that without the general information about temperature, humidity and geography, her descriptions might be less effective in evoking in us a feeling of what it is like to be surrounded by that white iciness.

Another way of thinking about these two approaches is to consider Miss Smilla's idiographic account as an artistic one, where the personal beauty and terror of the experience is paramount, and more general information about snow is sacrificed to the evocative narrative; whereas more general information belongs to science, logic and 'objective' truth, capturing qualities of snow that transcend the unique or peculiar.

This way of considering events rather polarises these two positions – of art and science – which is not necessarily in the best interests of music therapy. However, before attempting to reconcile these fields, and to consider music therapy and music psychology in relation to them (as separate or as interwoven), it may be useful to remind ourselves of the divide between the arts and the sciences that is our inheritance from the Renaissance Period in Europe.

Art and Science

The Renaissance gave rise to the mechanistic, and later the materialist, view of life and the positivist approach to science. Prior to the Renaissance, the arts and the sciences were interwoven in a human view of the world that was dominated by Aristotle's ideas. These influenced Western thinking, as well as Islamic thought, and were consonant with thinking on the Chinese and Indian continents. Aristotelian knowledge was based on the evidence of the senses, and matter and mind – or form and matter – were seen as being interdependent in a dynamic interrelationship. René Descartes is usually scapegoated as the instigator of the mind–body split (and the separation of art and science), and the conceptualisation of the human body (and for that matter, the universe), as being governed by mathematical law. Thus the body began to be understood as being made up of parts that could be taken apart and examined, rather like parts of a lawn mower or a sewing machine. The mind could be separated from the body; and spiritual life began to be seen as transcending physical life, where they had always been seen as one. This gave rise to what theologians came to call 'hierarchical dualism', where, in theological terms, spiritual matters came to be seen as superior to the physical realm. From the scientific perspective, of course, the reverse became true – and has only recently been re-examined, especially in the realm of quantum physics.

Descartes was not alone: Francis Bacon went further than Descartes in asserting that the role of science was not simply to understand the universe, but to exercise control over it; and Galileo Galilei believed that matter had to be studied only in its quantitative aspects: matter needed to be measured objectively and understood mathematically. Isaac Newton created an understanding of the universe as a system of interconnected, concrete objects moving in space. These developments had profound influences on human thought, and had direct consequences on art and music. Science became the dominant world view, seeking to measure and control nature, and the arts became a separate and distinctive discipline, allocated to the less rational realm of human experience. By the end of the 19th century, there was an overwhelming sense of security in the knowledge that science (and technology) could account for everything, although the Expressionist movement in art counteracted the social and personal effects of increasing industrialisation by emphasising their commitment to the heart and the human spirit (Aldridge *et al.* 1990). As we reach the end of the 20th century, there is still an emphasis on, and dominance of, science and logic in formal education, while Keynesian economics (which measure and quantify 'wealth' in standardised units) dominates global economic structures. The arts remain underfunded, and relegated to a 'specialist' and 'separate' area of knowledge.

It is within this context that we situate the emergence of Freud's ideas. His understanding of the Unconscious was based on the mechanistic model of the human body, translated into dynamic forces of the ego, id and superego that resembled physical energy. His view of human experience was embedded in a model of the psyche that was rational and objective, and that provided a structure within which individual and idiosyncratic human experience could be understood. Within the mechanistic context, we can understand the emergence of behavioural psychology, which identifies, quantifies and predicts human behaviour, and the development of cognitive psychology, which uses the computer as a metaphor for the brain and brain processes. It makes sense, therefore, that within this framework the world around us can be conceived as 'perceptual units' or 'units of information' that the brain groups, organises and co-ordinates into a system of information, much in the same way that music is broken up into what Leonard Meyer has called 'atomistic units' (Meyer 1994), i.e., units of rhythm, melody, pitch and so on, in order to understand how we perceive any one or all of these.

The language of science and objectivity, of logic and rationality, has dominated our thinking for hundreds of years. Within this mode, we, the 'observers', remain detached and objective when we describe and observe, much in the way that Freud remained detached and objective – scientific even – in listening to his patient's highly personal experiences.

But, as Stephen Mitchell (1993) articulates, there are moves afoot: we no longer, at a mass level, believe that science, technology and reason provide meaning that is personally – idiosyncratically – meaningful. We no longer believe that we can remain outside, and apart from, that which we seek to understand and describe fully. The 'new' science itself remains ungraspable and out of reach, and Danah Zohar (1991) suggests that our thinking is so fixed in Newtonian physics, that it is hampering us from making the major shift in thinking needed to grasp fully the new physics.

Stephen Mitchell sums up the revolution in thinking that is taking place, thus:

> As our understanding of the nature and limitations of scientific investigation changed, so has the place of science within western culture in general been transformed... In the postmodernism revolution in thought that has pervaded all the major intellectual disciplines, all knowledge, including scientific knowledge, is regarded as perspectival, not incremental; constructed, not discovered; inevitably rooted in a particular historical and cultural setting, not singular and additive; thoroughly contextual, not universal and absolute (Mitchell 1993, p.20).

This new thinking allows us to revisit music therapy from a position that need not take sides, so to speak, with either art or with science, but that allows us to develop a way of understanding the clinical work within its own context. This is both scientific and artistic, rather than being either artistic or scientific. Moreover, it would seem that a part of each of these traditions belongs to a 'universal' artistic/scientific tradition of music and therapy, and a part belongs to the highly personal and idiosyncratic.

Music therapy engages with 'art' not as a luxury, nor as fine art, nor as art that is removed from everyday experience. Rather, as David Aldridge (1991, 1993a) reminds us, both art and science together are necessary to portray and express the life of human beings. In considering the 'art of healing' (as in its parallel, the 'science of healing'), we are reminded to combine rigour with imagination – and it is this rigour and imagination that

I hope to emphasise in the following discussions – dialogues between music psychology and music therapy.

But first, we might ask ourselves why we need to engage at all with music psychology. Do music therapists need to know these concepts and insights?

The demand for more rigorous thinking by music therapists is not new. For too long, access to the professional literature has been complicated (and somewhat undermined) by, at one end of the spectrum, highly personal and unsystematic accounts of music therapy that do little to enhance the profession's status; and, at the other extreme, glamorous number crunching and attempts at standardised and 'objective' truth that seem to have little bearing on the dynamic, live and idiographic experience in the music therapy room. In between the two, accounts need to be systematic and rigorous, and accessible to the 'scientific', the 'artistic' and the 'therapeutic' communities. I see an exploration into music psychology as an attempt at pausing, and at enriching our understanding and our explanations of the musical act in music therapy.

Moreover, I am increasingly dissatisfied with what appears to be an emerging dichotomy between 'qualitative' and 'quantitative' research approaches (Wheeler 1995) and, while music therapy research falls outside the scope of this book, there is an undertow that suggests, tacitly, that qualitative research may have closer links with music therapy as an 'art', and quantitative research with music therapy as a 'science'.

If we continue to think of 'art' and 'science' as mutually exclusive, then music therapy is not going to be accommodated, with any comfort, by either camp. Neither idiographic nor monothetic accounts do full justice to the practice. Lesley Bunt (1994) has challenged music therapists to consider a synthesis between art and science, in which we think not so much of objective or subjective writing, but rather think with a subjectivity that is not too personal or idiosyncratic and that is sufficiently rigorous – and imaginative – to convey objectivity that is alive and convincing.

Although music therapists on the whole are not especially interested in the cognitive or perceptual functioning of clients – unless, of course, they are assessing these very aspects – it seems that we take for granted the mechanics of what is, after all, a fascinating and complex musical event. Clients, who are usually not musicians, are involved in what may be complex musical acts without 'knowing' what they are doing. Music therapists exercise a range of complex skills as part of music therapy improvisation. At the basic or natural level, the therapist and client function perceptually in how they receive auditory information, and organise it in a way that makes sense to them. Their musical acts indicate the use of auditory memory and transfer of information to motor responses, and these movements are defined and limited by the shape and size of the instruments being played. Moreover, a subtle and very quick inter-cueing takes place between the players, who have different levels of cognitive skills, in order to generate a musical whole.

Music Psychology

Much of the perceptual and cognitive psychology of music literature fits into the realm of the objective, quantitative and rational world view – although we must be careful not to ignore that aspect of the discipline that is qualitative and highly descriptive – and no less rigorous for this methodology. Much of the music psychology literature explored in the next two chapters deals with over-specific and reductionistic aspects of musical experience. The theories drawn from these tiny or reductionistic aspects of musical experience can be tedious to music therapists, many of whom experience – and generate – the idiosyncratic aliveness of music in its totality – but this is no reason to ignore the literature.

Music therapists are not alone: musicians, too, struggle with music psychology literature, and according to Rita Aiello (1994), musicians have been known to be careless in interpreting psychological experiments on musical experience. This carelessness highlights an inherent problem for musicians – and, I suggest, for music therapists – in coming to grips with aspects of music psychology. Much perceptual and cognitive music psychology literature is based on experimental material that Aiello calls 'musically impoverished'. In other words, music psychologists might test the perception of melody by playing 'pure tone' melodies produced by a synthesiser. This melody needs to be devoid of any rhythmic form, dynamic variation, change in timbre and so on, in order to ensure that these other aspects of music do not interfere with establishing how we perceive melody. Including the rhythmic form or dynamic variation would, invariably, affect how we hear the melody. Methods of enquiry such as these are based on the mechanistic view of matter: i.e., that by taking apart global phenomena and examining their fragments, we gain a detail and depth that contributes to the understanding of the whole, once the parts are reassembled. Musicians have a different rigour that would strongly resist compartmentalising music into rhythm, pitch, dynamic level and timbre, but that encompasses all of these as being part of music.

I suspect that music therapists share musicians' sentiments, in the sense that music, in all its multi-faceted dimensions, is the tool with which we practise our craft. The key issue for music therapists is whether the literature on music psychology, which combines rigorous thinking with systematic enquiry, has any practical application to music therapists who are primarily clinicians, 'in the (complex and unpredictable) field', with little time to read papers which seem to have little direct bearing on their work. Is this a reason to ignore 'scientific' literature? As practitioners who may feel more comfortable in the 'arts', do we, perhaps, need to broaden our enthusiasm and become more accepting and receptive to abstracted, reductionistic and generalised truths?

Finally, despite the focus of interest for music therapists being the richness of meaning that happens *between* the therapist and client in an *interpersonal* rather than in an *intermusical* sense, the medium through which the interpersonal is 'read' and 'decoded', so to speak, is a musical one. The next chapters explore aspects of music psychology in the belief and hope that it will broaden and enrich the framework within which music therapists describe their work – and that music psychologists may themselves be inspired by this enquiry.

CHAPTER 5

Perception, Cognition and Improvisation[1]

An American friend, who is a respected performer of contemporary piano music, visited me in Scotland and was fascinated by the musical content of audio tapes of some clinical work. On impulse I suggested that she improvise at the piano in a manner that supported my spontaneous drumbeats (i.e., that she be the 'music therapist'). There was no time to theorise about how to do this, but since she is skilled in playing highly complex rhythmic and arrhythmic structures, I assumed that this would be straightforward. I began to play on a conga drum in a fairly restrained and predictable manner, anticipating that she would meet and match me musically. Her rather sluggish textures puzzled me. It was not that they were 'wrong' musically, but rather that I felt unmet. I could not quite understand why this should be. Looking back on that event, it would seem that my musician friend was not 'tuning in' to me. I had – rather naively – assumed that since she was a proficient pianist, and since she knows me well, she would easily be able to hear and acknowledge me in the music.

The above scenario highlights the particular acuity exercised by music therapists immersed in a musical event that involves listening to another and to one's self, generating music that is congruent with what one hears, appropriate for both oneself and for the other, and assigning therapeutic as well as musical meaning to this spontaneous, jointly created event.

While the complexities of the therapeutic event cannot fully be explained by the language of perception and cognition, which is the language of this chapter, the discourse of music therapy often bypasses, and makes assumptions about, the very essence of the improvisation event. If we dissect the first moments of improvising with a client, we see that, as music therapists, we listen first of all to the spontaneous sounds made by clients on whichever instruments they play. As we listen, we organise these sounds in our minds using natural perceptual brain mechanisms so that these sounds become

---

1   I am grateful to Jane Davidson for her comments on this, and the following, chapter.

ordered and grouped into patterns. By creating patterns in our minds we begin to discern sequential groupings; and, at the same time, we assign these sounds with musical meaning – i.e., we do not hear a string of sounds, but rather we hear music. This musical meaning is learnt: it is part of our cultural conditioning, and it is part of our training as musicians and as music therapists. As the client continues to improvise, we continue to receive – and to perceive – new sound cues from them, and we begin to generate music, spontaneously and tentatively at first, in a way that seems to fit most appropriately with the sounds that the client is generating. In doing this, we are portraying the client's sounds in a particular musical style. As we play with the person, our memory strings together the sounds that we are playing and the sounds that they are playing concurrently, and while continuing to respond to musical cues from the client through our motor activity of playing music, a musical structure begins to take shape in our minds. We begin to shape our contribution to the joint improvisation with this structure in mind, conveying this information from our minds to our hands, at whichever instrument we are playing.

However, the interactive nature of the event means that we cannot simply impose our structure on what both of us are doing, concurrently. While creating music with the client, something the client does might, at any moment, result in a shift in the overall structure that we are creating in our minds as we listen and play: we might continue to shape the joint music, weaving in variations and shifts, in whichever stylistic idiom and structural form evolve as we continue to respond to musical cues from the client.

We might say that these skills are not unusual, in the sense that most improvising musicians possess them. What *is* unusual, in music therapy improvisation, is that it is not the music *per se* that dictates the direction of the improvisation, but rather how we are experiencing the client through the music that we play. This direct experiencing of the client – and of the client in relation to ourselves – through music, generates direct emotional communication between therapist and client. In music therapy improvisation, the learnt musical content, the stylistic and structural dictates take second place to the interpersonal meaning.

However, it is the music itself that portrays the emotional relationship, and this creates a paradox in meaning: the music generates and portrays the therapeutic relationship (some music therapists would say that it portrays *aspects* of the relationship), and yet to speak only in musical discourse does not convey the essence, and significance, of the relationship. To some extent here the paradox is ignored, since later chapters will address the non-musical mechanisms of music therapy improvisation.

Music therapists often take for granted, and do not question, basic perceptual mechanisms and cognitive processes intrinsic to the act of improvising. And yet without these events, no music-therapeutic relationship could take place.

In the opening scenario, my friend was a highly skilled musician who lacked therapeutic skills and could therefore not generate an interpersonal improvisation with me. In music therapy improvisation, clients are usually non-musicians. Unless they have suffered neurological injuries, music therapists assume that clients have intact perceptual mechanisms which enable them to create order out of the sounds that they make, both alone and with the therapist. Is this assumption correct? Moreover, clients usually lack the music-cognitive skills to assign musical meaning to the sounds created, even if their perceptual mechanisms are intact. How can we be sure that clients' experiences are not of noise that is dispersed and confusing? Also, in working with brain-injured patients, how can we tell that these clients actually form patterns from the sounds that they hear? In short, how can we be sure that clients hear – and experience – the music as music, and not as noise?

Music and Non-Music

Psychologists tell us that we are all able to distinguish between music and non-music, irrespective of whether we have musical knowledge or not. This seems a self-evident and rather banal statement, and yet, on thinking about it, I remember that although I know nothing about acting technique, whenever I switch on the television I instantly know (without hearing any sound) whether the person on the screen is 'acting' (i.e. portraying a character) or whether they are speaking 'as themselves' (e.g. in a documentary or news clip). Since we know that the basic perceptual processes are transferable between the visual and auditory senses, this analogy may help us to reflect on what distinguishes music from non-music.

For example, there is no way that the extraordinary varied palette of traffic sounds in downtown Johannesburg, with its incessant short bursts of hooting by roving taxis, bicycle bells, shouts of vendors and general street hubbub, could be experienced as music – and yet one might say that all the ingredients are there: the hooting has a rhythmic (or arrhythmic) quality that is at once predictive and unpredictive, the bicycle bells have a punctuating flavour, the shouts and conversations have melodic contours, and there are swells and dips of dynamic levels, sudden accellerandos of loud sounds, surprising silences, and so on. But the whole does not quite hold together.

If we transfer back to the sense of vision, it seems that in (mediocre) acting, the person's features do not tell one coherent story since there is a discrepancy in the various expressive modalities. For example, the intensity of the smile may be too strong for the more relaxed tone of the body, the timing of movements may be out of synchrony with the rhythm of the speech, and so on. The global impression of these conflicting messages enables me to detect instantly the degree of 'authenticity' of the person on the screen. In the same way, a lot of noises do not portray music for us. Rather we hear a whole tableau of disordered, disparate noises which do not make an integrated whole.

Some composers in the 1950s, of course, used precisely these kinds of sound in their compositions, attempting to find 'musical' applications for mechanical and everyday noises. Pierre Schaeffer named this music form 'musique concrete'. However, a distinction between 'noise that is noise' and 'noise that is art' may be that 'artistic' noise is endowed with artistic form: the composer 'does' something with it, rather than the 'noise' playing itself, so to speak. Thus composers of musique concrete might record sounds, and then accelerate the sounds, slow them down, remove and add certain frequencies, splice the tapes, and so on. This process of re-organising 'noise' transforms it towards 'art'. Another aspect to consider is whether 'noise is noise' simply because it is heard in the street and, therefore, do we say that 'noise is art' when we hear it in the concert hall? Or, as a *Guardian* reader puts it: 'How could I get an art gallery to purchase (at great expense) a mundane household object (e.g. an egg cup) from me? Would I have to go to art school first, or would I just have to say that the egg cup represented life and the universe?' (Notes & Queries, *The Guardian*, 29 May 1996).

As both Stravinsky and John Blacking inform us, though from very different positions, music is humanly organised sound. A person (or a group) creates sounds which have internal coherence, no matter how obscure, and this consistency is what we perceive instantly and use to identify music, whether we are musicians or not. This process is part of basic perceptual brain mechanisms. But something more needs to happen: perceptual mechanisms enable us to detect, and assign order to, external stimuli. These, however, need to become 'music', rather than remaining 'ordered sounds'.

As a music therapist, I have had the bewildering experience of adult clients who report, after a musically coherent improvisation, that the music sounds like 'a lot of noise' or 'a lot of nonsense'. How are they hearing the music? *Are* they hearing the music? Do they hear themselves in the music, and is this the 'nonsense' on which they are commenting? How does this idea that we 'perceive' consistency – or rather that perception enables us, quite immediately and naturally, to create order – fit with hearing and experiencing oneself in the music? This concept of hearing the self in the music is not peculiar to music therapy. John Blacking (1973, 1987) and John Shepherd (1991) take this concept a step further when they suggest that music reflects not just the self, but the self as part of a social structure. 'Social' music, according to their view, portrays the patterns and structures of society in music. Enculturated listeners recognise these in the music.

Leaving aside, for the moment, what it is that clients are conveying when they refer to the music as 'noise', which may be a metaphor for how they experience themselves in the world, it seems that we can be fairly assured that clients recognise the sounds as music, rather than as being 'not music'.

The next question, then, is this: do non-musician clients create, hear – and respond – to music as being made up of different ingredients, or are they creating, hearing and responding to one distinctive aspect of music, for example, that of rhythm, or melody, timbre, etc.?

Music as a Whole

It seems that when we listen to music, we hear it as a whole, rather than as disparate elements of rhythm, pitch, timbre, dynamic level, and so on. As we shall soon see, our minds are naturally predisposed to patterning. We can hold abstract patterns in our minds and adapt these with great flexibility in order to perceive and organise isolated and arbitrary musical events as coherent global experiences. In other words, we do not hear arbitrary, isolated sounds but group them together into a global experience. This is much in the same way as, in everyday communication, we receive information about the whole person, rather than isolating their eyes from their voice from their vocal timbre: we hear – and receive – a total, integrated soundscape. Indeed I suspect that it is only when there is a discrepancy between various modalities that we might think something like, 'only this person's mouth smiled, but not their eyes' or, 'what a noisy place'. In listening to the *total* event we are able to become aware of the absence of internal coherence; we then distinguish between music and non-music.

This idea of global perception gains support from the work of neuro-psychologists, Botez, Botez & Aube (1983) and Roederer (1982), all of whom make a case for the brain's capacity to experience music 'holistically'. According to them, musical sound form activates our inborn neural networks, i.e., it is not just the rhythm or the melody or the timbre that triggers specific parts in isolation from one another. Thanks to the complex inter-functioning of the brain, it seems that we are capable of perceiving music as holistic in nature, rather than as being made up of disparate elements. Indeed when music is used to treat neurological diseases, it is the whole of music that is used, not one aspect of it. Aldridge (1993b) reports, for instance, on the use of music to treat brain-injured patients who suffer from an aphasic speech disorder, and describes that it is the inflection, pitch and rhythm in the melodies that stimulate patients towards breathing and singing. The global music processing strategies of the brain are stimulated by music, and this global effect addresses and influences those parts of the brain that are malfunctioning.

Most of this makes perfect sense to music therapists: it confirms our intuition that clients – whether neurologically intact or not – have an experience of music as a 'whole', despite, for the most part, being musically naive. Even when clients whose neurological functioning is intact report that the music sounds like 'noise', they are referring to the whole being 'noisy' rather than one aspect of it. Unless, of course, they refer to the particular sound quality of an instrument. Even here, when a client reports finding the sound of, for example, the metallophone, disturbing, it is often necessary to clarify whether it was the music that we played which was the problem or whether, in fact, the client has a sensitivity to the timbre of that particular instrument. In talking about the improvisation, clients will identify a 'slow bit' or a 'lively' or 'quiet bit', in other words, they are identifying the music of that particular section as *a whole* – its overall flavour is slow, quiet or lively or whatever. It would seem, then, that as humans we do not distinguish between the rhythm, timbre or dynamic level of an improvisation, much as when we recall a conversation with someone we recall its totality. We recall what they said, how it was said, and probably also how we responded at the time. These are interlinked, and we would find it difficult to separate (robot-like) the texture of someone's voice from the semantic content – unless we were carrying out linguistic analysis.

It is, however, precisely at the more detailed level of analysis of the session (usually after the session has ended) that music therapists may choose to examine moments in the session at a purely musical level. We may have noted a particular excerpt from the tape recording of the session because something significant happened in the session at that moment, that we need to analyse in detail. Here our cognitive musical faculties are involved. For instance, we may contextualise the improvisation within a stylistic framework: we think about its metrical, rhythmic, harmonic components, as well as its overall flavour of tension and resolution, momentum, and so on. We may, in addition, reproduce this by singing a melody or trying out a harmonic sequence on an instrument, in order to grasp what we did spontaneously in the session and possibly develop it further. This complex and sophisticated process is beyond the natural mechanisms of human perception that order sounds into patterns. As musicians, we have learnt various 'grammars' of musical styles, we know how to reproduce the grammar that we have in mind; we know how to improvise and develop it; and we also know how to switch grammars suddenly, without the therapeutic improvisation losing its sense of wholeness.

However, none of these musical cognitive processes would occur without our basic perceptual functioning, which may be seen as a lower level of processing information, in the sense of being almost pre-meaningful. We need to order sounds into patterns and groups before our cognitive functioning can assign musical meaning to basic perceptual forms.

It is at this level of reflection of the session – a level that focuses on the musical content and isolates the 'musical' aspect – that the concepts offered by music psychology may be useful frameworks for us to think about and describe the therapeutic medium through which music therapists work – that of music. I now explore various perceptual mechanisms that are activated when we listen to music; whether we listen during the act of improvising with clients or whether we listen to recordings of sessions.

Perceptual Grouping Mechanisms

Grouping mechanisms are fundamental to perceptual processes: without these the world would be a 'buzzing booming' mass that made no sense whatsoever. For more detail, I refer readers to the writings of Deutsch (1982), Serafine (1988), Dowling and Harwood (1986), Sloboda (1985) and others. These descriptions of grouping mechanisms help us to understand how a particular musical element is perceived in relation to its local context. For example, an isolated note or sound is meaningless: it gains meaning when we perceive its relationship with other notes – what has preceded it, where it fits in the context of the total phrase, what its tempo relation is to other notes, and so on. These relationships to other notes or beats are created by our minds instantly: in other words, we organise the sounds that we hear into perceptual structures directly through our sensory systems, and this is a 'natural' rather than a 'learnt' process. Thus as a music therapy client begins to play the first few notes or beats on a drum, we integrate the local events, as they occur, almost instantaneously. However, as the client continues to play, and, perhaps, we join in, the broader structure of an improvisation is dependent upon our recall of earlier perceptions – i.e., of the opening beats – and our capacity to integrate these with new perceptions as they occur – this is not necessarily a sequential process, but rather a kaleidoscopic one where each new piece of information changes our perception of the whole. As new local events are generated, we perceive them, our musical memory recalls earlier events, and our brain receives and organises them in terms of local features. The musical meaning that we assign to them, is a cognitive, rather than perceptual, process, which will be addressed later.

In terms of our perceptual mechanisms, psychologists have isolated the following basic perceptual mechanisms of the brain.

The horizontal and vertical structure of music

Depending on our attentional stream, when we listen to music we focus on the momentum of sound patterns either vertically (chord sequences) or horizontally (following a melody or distinguishing between a lower or higher melodic line). We cannot, perceptually, focus on both the vertical and the horizontal pattern of a piece, although we experience them as co-existing.

The Gestalt principles

The Gestalt principles of grouping mechanisms were first developed by psychologists primarily in terms of the visual senses. More recently, music psychologists have transferred these principles to how we perceive sound stimuli: how we create patterns out of what we hear, how we decide what goes together, where there are disjunctions, what is included and excluded, and so on.

When we listen to music, we group together notes that follow a common rule, for example, the continued ascent of a scale, the repetition of a single note, or notes that move in the same direction: we perceive these as belonging together, rather than as separate, isolated events. This is known as the principle of *good continuation*.

We also group together musical elements such as time or pitch, which are close to each other, i.e., the closer together two sounds or stimuli, the more likely we are to hear them as belonging together temporally. Thus when we hear sounds whose spacing is ** ** ** **, we hear ** as belonging together, rather than grouping together the end of one group and the beginning of the next, i.e. *(* *)*. Where there is no obvious dimension such as pitch or rhythm to group sounds together, we group together sounds with similar timbre. Dowling and Harwood (1986) report that cultures across the world give preferences to smaller intervals over larger intervals within their tonal systems, and this, they suggest, is derived from the physiological structure of the ear. Indeed the violation of proximity is used, in Western and non-Western music, for aesthetic effect.

We group together events into regular rather than irregular sequences or chords (this is the principle of *regularity*); and the grouping principle of *symmetry* describes our preference for symmetrical rather than asymmetrical groups. Here psychologists suggest that the perceived simplicity of nursery tunes is that they are divisible successively and symmetrically into even numbers of groups of notes. We know that symmetry, like regularity, is a basic principle of stability.

Finally, the grouping together of sounds that are similar, rather than different, is the principle of *similarity*: visually, the principle is illustrated in Figure 5.1. In terms of vision, we perceive four vertical rows, rather than horizontal lines, because we group together the stars and the circles.

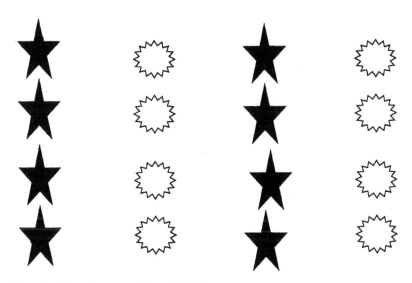

Figure 5.1 Visual representation of similarity

Higher order groups

We form higher order groups by combining together groups formed by any of the above factors. Thus notes are grouped together into a phrase, and several phrases might be grouped together into a cluster of phrases over a section of a piece of music. Chords might be grouped together to give us a harmonic progression, or beats and off-beats are grouped together by their repetitiveness and similarity.

All of these are fundamental, and instant, perceptual events which have to do with any sound stimuli, whether musical or not. How these sound events become musically meaningful is a result of cognitive processes, which I explore below, focusing on two concepts: those of schema theory and invariants.

Schemata

One way of considering how we make sense of the world is to think in terms of mental schemata. Schemata can be described as knowledge structures that we develop from early childhood in the course of living in, and learning about, the world. In terms of music, we develop schemata by hearing many of our culture's melodies from infancy: schemata are a way of representing the structure of a piece of music. In music, schemata may be thought of as being temporal, in the sense that they guide our expectations as to what happens next in a piece of music, what we attend to and what we remember. Lerdahl (1991) suggests that schemata are based on simple configurations to do with basic principles of stability, such as, for example, phrase symmetry or a harmonic progression such as I–IV–V–I, which, as we have learnt, offers a sense of completion. These relatively simple configurations are easily learnable, become part of our long-term memory and have the potential to influence our cognitive organisation of new stimuli.

According to schema theory, we organise experience into structured categories. In listening to music, experienced listeners already have access to the basic schema of a piece, such as the introduction, coda, antecedent and consequent phrases, and knowledge of this schema guides our understanding and expectation of how the piece will develop. The schema is projected forward, generating expectations as to what comes next (Lerdahl 1991). The interruption of an ongoing schema brings about physiological arousal: our sense of habituation is interrupted, and what follows is a cognitive activity that searches for meaning as to what has happened, and an integration of the new and interuptive event into a new meaningful pattern for the piece.

At the same time, experienced listeners have access to certain features of musical style: we can think of style as being the features or principles shared by a group of compositions, for example a particular combination of rhythm, melody, harmony, and phrasing. According to Meyer's information theory, it is the interruption of our expectations, or the deviation from an expected stylistic development, that causes aesthetic pleasure in experiencing music.

Comments on listening to music

It would seem that the process of listening to a piece of music is complex, and that what we, as listeners, make of a piece of music is the result of a constant reappraisal of what is happening in the music. As we have seen, in listening we use perceptual grouping mechanisms in order to organise sounds into local patterns, which we then identify as fitting together into higher ordered groupings. At the same time, through our experience of the world, we have access to the schema structures, which enable us to identify the overall structure of a piece of music, and to recognise, and take pleasure in, deviations from this plan. As well as the structural plan, there are certain stylistic features (e.g. the tango rhythmic, the 7th chord in blues, a harmonic structure used by Romantic composers) that we recognise as being a particular musical grammar found in one piece or across several pieces that we group together as belonging to a musical style.

These 'proto-typical' features can be removed from a particular style and transferred to another. We recognise these 'cognitive reference points' through familiarity across different musical styles: thus we recognise a tango rhythm, for example, in Stravinsky's 'The Soldier's Tale', despite the harmonies not being those of the Latin American idiom. Lee (1991) speaks of ambiguous music, which he calls 'ungrammatical' – i.e., music that departs from a coherent musical grammar: this music may share features of different schemata, and we synthesise the various schemata, and create new ones for ourselves, through a process of 'perceptual reconstruction' – i.e., adding and subtracting features that are already familiar to us. Cognitive psychologists would agree with Leonard Meyer (1973), often thought of as the father of cognitive psychology, who suggests that it is this process of new synthesis that is part of the pleasure of listening to, and experiencing, music.

Finally, in listening to music we may think of an ongoing process of perception and cognition, as the music unfolds. Psychologists Robert West, Peter Howell and Ian Cross (1985) explain that in listening to music, we identify, '…what elements go together, where disjunctions occur, and inclusion of elements and groups of elements in superordinate groups. It also requires identification of elements perceived as structurally important, as opposed to those which are in some sense, embellishments' (p.44). They suggest that not only do we group similar or related musical elements together, but we are also able to order the groupings into higher and lower levels by identifying what is essential to the musical structure of a piece, and what is an elaboration of the essential. For example, a musical phrase would be a higher level, made up of rhythmic forms, melodic sections, and so on, and a rhythmic cluster would be a lower structural level.

Comments on grouping mechanisms, schema theory
My music therapist's intuition about the perceptual mechanisms described above is that they help music therapists to understand how we experience music, and how musically naive clients can make sense of the sounds that they – that we – are generating in the session. However, this is incomplete for music therapists. Just as my American friend, presumably perceptually

and cognitively intact, did not assign the 'right' meaning to the improvisation; and just as cognitive psychologists would say that simply to perceive is
not what gives meaning, but rather it is the knowing and the interruptions
of expectations that give meaning to the event, so music therapists would
say that perception and cognition – and emotion – do not suffice. Moreover,
music therapists are left with explaining why and how someone who is
neurologically intact but severely emotionally disturbed, describes 'noise'
and 'chaos' rather than musical sounds that make sense. In other words, can
emotional factors override perception? How do these concepts help us to
capture the improvisation's interactional – and interpersonal – significance?

In listening to recordings of music therapy sessions, it seems that music
therapists often work 'against' musical cognition in order to discern what is
going on interactively or interpersonally. In other words, music therapists
need to 'exit' learnt and trained musical cognitive processes in order to listen
beyond the music, so to speak. This does not mean that music therapists
listen non-perceptually', as in William James' 'buzzing and booming' confusion. Rather the music therapist's focus has a different strategy. When
hearing sounds, we group them as a result of 'natural' perceptual grouping
processes, but the therapeutic meaning that we assign the grouping, and the
interruption of generated musical expectations, is not explained in terms of
musical-cognitive processes. For example, a melody that is cognitively and
schematically compelling may be one that, as music therapists, we may at
times turn away from, in the interests of eliciting, meeting and responding
to the 'dynamic form' generated by the improvisation. As we shall see later,
dynamic form is elicited in therapeutic improvisation techniques that are
specifically activated in order to generate an emotional/therapeutic – rather
than a musical – relationship between therapist and client. Thus while a
melody may be musically compelling, and cognitively and schematically
congruent, the interests of dynamic form improvisation may result in the
music therapist turning away from its anticipated course. This, however, is
not for artistic effect. At other times we may need to ignore a more prominent
attentional stream in the interests of decoding the therapeutic communication and interaction.

This turning away from what is a cognitively determined listening bias,
developed as part of our cultural learning, is part of music therapy training
and practice. This turning away is one way of explaining the distinction
between the way that a music therapist listens and improvises with someone,
and the way that a musician might do so. In a collaborative project with
Sandra Brown, in which we took turns at improvising music together (1) as
music therapist and client, and (2) as musicians improvising together, we

found in analysing the tapes that when we were playing as therapists, it was not the music that dictated the improvisation, but how we experienced the other person, the client, in the music. As musicians, we found that we could 'play', literally and indulgently, allowing the spontaneously created music to emerge and develop and dictate the improvisation (Brown and Pavlicevic 1996).

What made my music therapy training so excruciating was learning to improvise 'clinically' rather than 'musically': this involved turning away from cognitive structures that, over years of formal musical training, had become associated with a certain (Western) musicianship, in order to meet and extend clients' expression of themselves in clinical work. In music therapy, clients' expressions might be fragmented, asymmetrical, highly irregular and quite unmusical. This unmusicality might be understood as a perceptual or a cognitive deficit, or as suggesting a lack of musical training. Assuming that there is no perceptual or cognitive dysfunction, music therapists would understand the 'musical disorder' not so much as an absence of musicality or of musical training, but rather as the client 'sounding their pathology'. This is borne out by work with clients who may have learning difficulties, have never had any musical training, and produce the most exquisitely shaped, balanced and 'musical' music. In contrast, music therapy improvisa-tion with highly trained musicians who are in the throes of a mental illness, such as a bipolar depression, may reveal musical utterances that are disor-dered and lacking in any sense of musicality.

As therapists, a clinical task is to meet this 'pathology', which is sounded through the joint improvisation. For a while, and especially in early stages of sessions, this may involve improvising exclusively on the client's terms, rather than on mutually negotiated musical terms, and here the therapist needs to remain in what I call a 'counter-cognitive' – and exceedingly uncomfortable – mode of music-making. Disorder, after all, does not come naturally.

Musical disorder that has an emotional basis, is quite a different experi-ence from that found in contemporary music (improvised or pre-composed), although both might be said to create a high level of cognitive dissonance, with many interruptions, with highly asymmetrical, ungrouped sounds. When my American friend could not quite meet my spontaneous playing on the conga drum, we could understand this in terms of her music cognition being challenged, but since she is a skilled musician this seems unlikely. It was at a personal level that she did not meet me.

Looking back on that event, I understand the amount of 'unlearning' that goes into music therapy training which, after a while, we take for granted –

indeed we might say that *clinical* schemata are generated in our music therapy training which differ subtly from *musical* schemata, even if the clinical/musical schemata are portrayed through music. These clinical schemata have non-musical components, to do with the process of therapy and of relationship: these are part of clinical improvisations with clients, which, to a highly skilled musician who knows little about music therapy, would be inaccessible, despite the fact that the therapeutic process takes place through the music improvisation. My musician friend was not 'tuning in' in any other way than a musical one, and this was not sufficient for me, playing as me, the person. I was not playing a musical motif, I was – rather naively, perhaps – playing myself.

We could say, therefore, that there exists a particular acuity that is the music therapist's: it is not exclusively musical, but neither is it exclusively psychological. Rather this acuity is an interface between the two, as explained by the concept of dynamic form, with the therapist reading the emotional content of the improvisation through the music, and responding to this content through the music.

Invariants

But let us get back to music cognition for a minute. Although the Gestalt grouping principles described earlier are useful for understanding how our minds organise local pattern in music, musicians and music therapists operate not just at this level of grouping, but at higher or more 'global' levels of organisation which, as discussed, may be thought of in terms of schemata. But what holds a piece together in the first place, enabling us to create a schema as it unfolds?

Psychologists Jay Dowling and Dane Harwood (1986) employ Gibson's concept of invariants. These provide a constant throughout a piece of music and can be seen as underpinning various 'local' patterns, enabling us to hear music as a continuous, unfolding event, rather than as various bits one after the other. Invariants remain constant even when local patterns change. Examples of invariants are the musical pulse which remains constant no matter how complex the rhythmic or phrasing; the key or tonal organisation of a piece; or the instrumentation and density of sound texture that, despite fluctuations, remain constant.

Invariants may be highly implicit – for example, the pulse of a piece of music may be extremely subtle, and here we need to be able to listen beyond the surface structure of music in order to apprehend invariant structures that are considerably complex. The more complex – and more subtle – invariants are apprehended as a result of musical training and familiarity. For example, the invariant of pulse or periodicity is a basic one that any human being taps into, and this is more than likely the result of our being pulsating, periodic and cyclical beings. Thus a naive listener might listen to a Bach fugue as a foot-tapping experience or an invarient of pulse, while a more sophisticated listener will hear more complex invariants of harmonic style, tonalities and their modulations, of rhythmic clusters and so on.

Invariants may be specific to that particular piece (Dowling and Harwood quote the example of the melodic/rhythmic contour of the opening of Beethoven's Fifth Symphony) or they may have to do with musical style: for example, rhythmic or harmonic characteristics of several pieces. Our com-prehension of global invariants of structure (for example, of sonata form, rondo form or the particular rhythmic qualities of a tango or a barcarole) guides our expectations when we hear music, and this helps us to process the musical events as they occur over time. The music may match our expectations according to our understanding of the invariants for that piece, be they metrical, textual, stylistic or instrumental. In fact we could see invariants as providing a standard for evaluating moderate deviations from it. Conflicting invariants produce ambiguity and tension in the music, and this, Dowling and Harwood suggest, adds to the aesthetic enjoyment of a piece. This idea of interruption creating aesthetic tension is a tenet of Leonard Meyer's theory about how music generates emotion: it is the departure from our anticipations of where and when musical events will occur that generates feeling and emotion in the listener (Meyer 1956).

It seems that we need invariants to make sense of music, and if there is ambiguity in the music then we create our own invariants. We then hold these self-created patterns in our minds as a yardstick against which we hear the music. Lee (1985) shows that listeners try to establish the metre of a piece as soon as possible (often as soon as the third or fourth note), and tend to stick to this, despite later syncopations or ambiguities of metre.

Invariants and music therapy

The concept of invariants clarifies an aspect of clinical improvisation. First of all, in learning different harmonic densities, a range of rhythmic and arrhythmic motifs, we are learning how to assemble – and dissemble – potential clinical/musical invariants, for use in highly idiosyncratic improvi-sation. We learn to create chord progressions that have something in common, that hold together no matter how unconventionally; we learn to invert, extend, narrow chords, to play them in a manner that is pompous and grand, to play them tightly, playfully, narrowly, and so on, while at the same time retaining the essential quality of those chordal textures. All this gives us a vocabulary of different musical/emtoional invariants that enable us to be ready to match, meet, reflect, through the music improvisation, whatever clients do, and however musically/emotionally limited, fragmented, incoherent or confusing this might be.

The concept of invariants also helps to clarify how our (musically naive) clients' perceptions of the music may differ from our (musically sophisticated) own, despite, say, a highly mutual musical interplay in clinical improvisation. If the forming of perceptual groupings is indeed a 'natural' phenomenon (natural does not mean that the process of groupings is innate, but that we learn it naturally, through our exposure to the world), then musically naive clients who are neurologically intact can 'create' their own invariants, and although these may not be the same as the therapist's invariants, the two will 'fit' in the music. The concept of invariants also clarifies why musically sophisticated music therapy clients can be difficult to engage through clinical improvisation: their 'musical mindset' is fixed on the more conventional musical idioms. My experience of having musicians as clients is that there is some difficulty in separating making music for music's sake (according to conventional styles) and making music in order to 'sound themselves'.

As music therapists, we can also use the concept of invariants to help describe the *musical* manifestations of mutual communication between therapist and client: for example, we can think in terms of a fully mutual clinical improvisation as one where therapist and client generate invariants *together*. This is especially true in the opening moments of the improvisation, where there is a delicate interplay, with the therapist receiving one or two notes from the client, joining in responsively and flexibly, which means that the client's change of tempo allows for the invariant to be malleable, explored, before it is 'set'.

When the client appears impervious and 'deaf' to the therapist, playing compulsively and in a way that does not take the therapist into account, and the therapist is mainly in responsive mode, following the client, we could say that the client alone is setting the invariants – she or he is calling the tune. In this instance, the therapist perceives the invariants in the client's playing, recognises them and reflects them in her responsive playing with the client.

When improvising with a client's fragmented and highly disordered playing, the therapist first needs to experience the disorder as an invariant, i.e., the invariant is one of 'disorder'. The therapist may then offer a basic beat in the interest of creating a relationship. The basic beat is an invariant of 'order' – and this invariant needs to be congruent with the disordered invariant of the client. By sounding an ordered invariant, the therapist invites the client to hear his or her own (disordered) invariant against – or alongside – an ordered invariant which, somehow, fits in with the client's disorder. Now this is an apparently contradictory statement. If the client's playing is highly disordered, how can the therapist offer order that is *congruent with* the client's disorder, while *at the same time* meeting the client? We could describe this clinical skill in terms of invariants. As therapists, our listening is highly tuned to detecting order (or ordered invariants), even amid the extraordinary chaos that a 'fragmented' personality would display – which is itself an invariant. We then sift this fragile, latent order and reflect it to the client. Here I propose that if the 'order' is the 'correct' one (and if the client has the potential for integration), the client will move towards the ordered invariant, whereas if it is too far removed, or incongruent with the client's playing, the client remains isolated with his or her disordered invariant, and the therapist and client do not begin to move towards one another musically.

Another music therapy scenario is where there is too much confusion in the client's playing to enable the therapist to generate an invariant that is related to the chaotic invariant of the client. Here the therapist may need to create or invent an invariant of stability, and almost impose it, colonising the client's playing by imposing an order which is alien to it. Here, again, the created invariant of order needs, somehow or other, to be congruent with the client's invariant of chaos – and the therapist's clue as to whether it is congruent or not resides in the client's response to her offering the invariant.

A Final Note

Finally, in terms of perception and cognition, a key question remains: do music therapy clients need to be able to 'decode' the musical event in order to engage interpersonally within the improvisation? Do they need some awareness of the musical mechanisms in order to find the improvisation meaningful on an interpersonal level?

I suspect that music therapists would say that no, they do not need to make 'musical' sense of the music, since the focus of the improvisation is the interactive relationship; while cognitive psychologists might say that yes, they do, since it is what happens in the music that generates arousal and meaning. Without wanting to polarise the two positions, albeit hypothetically, music therapists need to be aware of the complexities of musical improvisation in music therapy. Do we really share meaning with clients in sessions? Is the therapist's meaning the same as the client's? If a client's experience is essentially non-musical, in that they do not 'understand' the music, is the total experience less musically meaningful to them? Does this absence or this diminished musical understanding detract from the inter-personal/emotional experience? Or does the inter-personal experience remain intact, despite the absence of musical insights? And finally, can we really separate the musical from the interactional experience in music therapy sessions? For the time being I would like to leave these questions unanswered.

CHAPTER 6

In Concert
Improvisation, Cognition and Music Therapy

Music improvisation has always been.

Before music was notated, oral tradition ensured that songs and pieces were kept alive through performance, and each performer added something distinctive to the music, which transformed it, albeit subtly. In Western music, the baroque era and early classical period were based on the improvisatory skills of the performers, with much music being notated only in terms of figured bass, which the performer 'filled in', so to speak. Improvisation in jazz is the order of the day, while 'serious' music has moved increasingly away from improvisation, as more and more aspects of performance are notated or else sealed on to electronic tape.

A substantial proportion of approaches to music therapy are based on music improvisation (Bruscia 1987), although there is a diversity in application in actual practice and in how the improvisation 'means'. In this section I explore improvisation from a perceptual and a cognitive position, with focus on Jeff Pressing's (1984, 1988) work which offers some useful concepts for understanding and explaining the inner mechanisms of music therapy improvisation.

However, whereas this literature assumes that the players are adept musicians, most music therapists improvise music with people who suffer from what we may broadly call 'disorders'. Some disorders affect basic perceptual processes, while others affect cognitive functioning. Any of these may interfere with the client's musical experience, whether at a level of listening, hearing, responding or playing. In addition, one of the difficulties of working with those who suffer from a mental illness is the complication of medication and its side effects. This may make it difficult to gauge whether such a patient's music is a reflection of their illness or of their medication. If the latter, it may be very difficult for the therapist to gauge whether the patient's disorganised or over-rigid playing can really be addressed. At a different level altogether is the work with patients suffering from senile dementia. Despite aspects of their brain clearly not functioning, grouping processes – and musical enjoyment – seem to remain intact. My own clinical experience is affirmed by the work of Aldridge (1993b) and that of Aldridge and Aldridge (1992) and Aldridge and Brandt (1991) and that is that many dementia patients are able to sustain a mutual and highly emotionally and musically satisfying interaction with the therapist, which inevitably diminishes as the patient's condition deteriorates. Although the discussion below is based on normal perceptual functioning it hopes to contribute to the discourse on music therapy improvisation.

Form

In their paper entitled 'Is Everyone Musical?', Sloboda, Davidson and Howe (1994) suggest that most members of a culture evolve receptive musical skills through casual exposure to the music of their culture. This enables even so-called 'non-musical' people in western culture to have some idea about how music is 'put together', even if they have neither the skill to perform it nor the language to describe it.

As musicians who are not only familiar with (culture-bound) musical structures, but also understand how music is constructed in terms of specific harmonic or melodic progressions, improvisers have the basis on which to embellish these structures. These improvised embellishments include, e.g., variations of existing melodies, adding passing notes and chords to what already exists, or moving away from a melodic/harmonic/rhythmic idiom before returning to it, as in a jazz riff or a set of improvised variations. What is it that dictates the improviser's decisions?

In a 'free' improvisation, we might say that the changes, deviations and delays are dictated by the player's need for change and, more excitingly perhaps, by the player's inventive use of musical 'errors'. The error provides a departure or a distraction, a departure that is exciting or pleasing and that may be developed. Here we are reminded of Leonard Meyer's Information Theory, discussed earlier, which states that it is the delay, variation and departure from established or known musical structure, and dips into 'ungrammatical' style, that heighten our state of arousal and emotional excitement.

Ansdell (1995) describes improvisation as being 'beyond right and wrong' and as having the 'space for the unexpected' (p.24). He describes Keith Jarrett's solo piano improvisation in which a 'wrong note' becomes absorbed into the music, creating a new direction for the improvisation, rather than the performer adhering to the harmonic and textural tone of the improvisation up to that moment. The development of the improvisation, by 'seizing the moment' alters and extends its formal structure, although an improviser of Jarrett's standing would still be able to maintain an overall view of the form as it unfolds.

In music therapy, we can consider the form of the music as being dictated, not by musical structural conventions, but rather by the emotional and relational dictates of the jointly created, therapeutic improvisation. Thus where the therapist experiences the client's music as being, for example, dispersed and difficult to pin down and relate to, the therapist might, in response to this, initiate a symmetrical, rather staid musical structure in order to provide a predictability and constancy for the client. This is an interpersonal, therapeutically informed improvisatory impulse, embodied through the musical act – and it gives rise to improvisatory form with therapeutic significance. The evolving musical structure is not only prescribed by the rather dispersed playing of the patient: in fact, were the therapist playing as only-musician, the musical form suggested by the client might be heard as loose and unsequential, possibly almost pointillistic in style. The *musical* response to this might create form more in keeping with the client's musical style. The therapeutic emphasis, however, may necessitate a structure that is rather staid within which to improvise – which may, in fact, be rather unmusical.

Referents

Pressing (1984) describes what he calls the improviser's 'referents'. These points of reference, so to speak, are central to the improvisation in that they provide the improviser with 'beacons' of orientation to which the improviser may return or remember while developing a new section of the improvisation. A referent may be a musical structure, a mood or a motive: it is the basis from which the improvisation departs and to which it returns. I understand the concept of referents to be parallel to that of invariants, described in the previous chapter, but on a broader scale – or higher level of grouping. Whereas invariants can be seen as lower levels of musical structure, such as, e.g., a pulse or a rhythmic pattern that enables us to hold the piece together in our minds, a referent may be a particular musical phrase or musical motif that the musician recognises and returns to, in free improvisation, as a point of reference.

The relationship between the referent and the improvisation is variable, and includes the use of imitation, canon, counterpoint and variation, in which the referent is constantly present; or the improvisation may be independent from the referent. Here only what Pressing calls 'free' or 'absolute' improvisation has no referents, with the music continuing to unfold in an unpredictable way that makes it difficult to refer back to what happened earlier in the piece.

In contrast to a solo improvisation, when an ensemble of musicians is improvising together, a more detailed and explicit referent is needed to, provide information for the players about their relationships, the timing of their various riffs, the moment at which they all return to the chorus, and so on. In a group improvisation, each player's own time-point sequence will interact with that of the other players: for example, the players will agree upon, or share a perception of, where and how phrases end, pauses occur, at what point they 'return to the fold', and so on. Pressing suggests that when there are no agreed upon referents between the players, they are playing in co-existing streams rather than interrelating musically. This brings to mind play in early childhood, which developmental psychologists describe as 'parallel' play, in which children play near to each other and may, at certain moments, use one another's toys, but they are essentially involved in their own games; contrasted with this is co-operative play, in which children together negotiate the games and their rules.

The idea of improvisational referents resonates strongly with music therapy improvisation. For example, in work with an adolescent boy, we together developed a musical sequence which he hummed quietly and shyly, as we improvised together at the piano. This sequence became a musical 'beacon', to which we would return time and again, after, in between, developing the improvisation in all kinds of different directions. The referent was not always played in the same way, but we always knew when we had found it. Indeed part of the pleasure, and part of its power, was recognising it within the opening chord, and of then expanding, shrinking, expanding or unravelling it as we wanted to.

Time Points

Pressing describes an improvisation as a sequence of musical events that are triggered at specific moments (which he calls time points) in the improvisatory process. Thus a new musical event may be triggered at the ends of musical phrases, at the end of grouped sequences and as a result of a pause or a cadence. The improviser makes the critical decision with regard to how and where these time points occur, and how the new sequence of musical events will develop.

In a spontaneous music therapy improvisation, where therapist and client are jointly creating the improvisation, rather than jointly improvising on a set musical theme, both the musical events and the time points are negotiated between the players, rather than being predetermined and/or being imposed by the therapist. As a result of her musical training, the therapist may (in her mind), expect a phrase to end at a certain point in terms of musical style. However, the client, who has no such musical conditioning, does not support this expectation. This then makes the therapist review where a phrase might end and a new musical cluster begin. This is part of the 'unlearning' that therapists undergo, alluded to earlier.

Another scenario, of course, is where the therapist directs the time points by presenting an improvisational structure which is fixed in her mind – and not negotiable: for example, the therapist might present an ostinato – a repeated pattern over which the client improvises. Here the ostinato is a steadying and containing structure: its repetition provides predictability and the client can begin to anticipate the therapist's musical movements. This provides the client with the opportunity to adapt her own playing in order to remain congruent with the therapist. A third scenario is where the therapist simply follows or supports the client's playing, which may meander with no perceptible point to define a preceding cluster. The music provides no beacon to demarcate a section and refer back, and so the therapist accompanies the client's meanderings. This has been a familiar scenario, especially when working with people suffering from chronic schizophrenia (Pavlicevic and Trevarthen 1989, 1994).

There is also the context of the client being over-organised and inflexible in their spontaneous playing: their repetition of, for example, a rhythmic pattern sets the time points in a fixed, rigid manner, and here the spontaneity of the interaction is threatened. In the same way that we would find talking to someone who said the same thing over and over again tedious and limiting in terms of getting to know that person, the therapist is constrained by the client's cramping boundaries, often not negotiable.

Redundancy

Each cluster of musical events in an improvisation contains aspects that are simultaneously valid and redundant, and the improviser(s) make split-second decisions as to what to use and what to discard as the improvisation unfolds. Each of these aspects, which are acoustic, musical and kinetic, as well as emotional and visual, exists in two forms: intended and actual. The intended form is triggered at specific time moments, with decisions made as to what is valid and what is redundant, and the corresponding actual form is constructed from memory of past musical events in the improvisation, how these are linked to preceding and subsequent events, and how the current event is unfolding in relation to the overall improvisation.

The gap between the intended and actual form reduces with training and practice. Figure 6.1 shows the factors that influence the size of the gap between the intended and the actual musical act. The axis x(1) shows that the higher the level of musical skill, the smaller the gap between the actual and intended form. With practice we are able to actualise more accurately what we intend (a), or what we hear in our minds. In contrast, a musically naive improviser's intentions may be actualised in a rather hit-and-miss manner (b). Axis x(2) shows that the more complex the music, the wider the gap (c) between actual and intended, and vice versa (d).

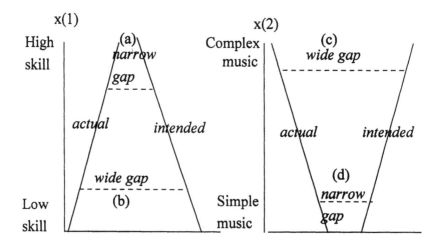

Figure 6.1 The gap between the actual and the intended musical act

In music therapy improvisation, two people with rather different levels of musical skill are together creating an improvisation. Each of their intentions and actualisations may have different 'size' or quality of gaps, and it seems that various kinds of gaps between actual and intended may be occurring simultaneously. For example, the client may not be able to actualise what she or he intends: a client may say something like, 'I know what I want to play but I don't know how to do it'. But at the same time, the (musically naive) client may be experiencing the improvisation at a lower level of cognition, one that is more accessible to his or her musical experience. For example, the client may be experiencing the improvisation purely at the level of periodicity or predictability, which in Figure 6.1 is (d). In other words, they are experiencing the music as 'simple', and here they can more or less actualise what they intend: the gap between intended and actual is small, even though the client has a low level of musical skill. At the same time, the therapist may be experiencing the same improvisation at a more complex level (c) of, say, harmonic structure, contrapuntal melodies, and so on – as well as, of course, the 'clinical' and interpersonal level – and here actualising the intention may be more complex, despite her high musical skill. Each player's intention and actual musical utterances occur in parallel, in co-operation and in tandem to one another, and the players may 'fit' musically and personally – while not necessarily coinciding cognitively – as a result of different degrees of musical experience and skill.

How can something that has different levels of meaning for each person, fit between them? It seems that each player reflexively (or pre-reflexively?) accommodates, to varying degrees, the intentions of the other person, as these are embodied through the musical sounds. Somehow or other, these two different experiences come together in music therapy to produce a single improvisation.

From a music therapy perspective, I would suggest that the degree to which the two players' improvisation fits has to do with the therapist's skill in accommodating the client's musical utterances, as well as the client's personal flexibility in being 'interpersonally available'.

Another gap between intended and actual depends on what 'musical' feedback the therapist receives from the client. Although it is somewhat contrived to separate the musical from the music-therapeutic, the musical *is* an aspect of the music-therapeutic and is the focus of discussion here. The therapist may have a musical intention which is congruent with the preceding joint playing. However, she may have to forego that in the interests of responding to the client's musical utterances, which may have, at that moment, different qualities to those the therapist had anticipated. The therapist often has to make split-second changes in gear (and crash into reverse gear if necessary) in the interests of 'being with' the client. Also, in therapeutic improvisation, the therapist is not exclusively in 'musician' mode, so that musical events that make musical sense become redundant in the interests of the therapeutic process. For example, from a musical perspective, the improvisation may be demanding a change of rhythm, pace, dynamic level or tonality; however, the therapist has to curb her musical 'aesthetic instinct' in the interests of the here-and-now of the therapeutic process, which may well demand that, for the time being, the music continues along the same lines.

In music improvisation, the improviser makes a choice between generating new event clusters which have associations of similarity or contrast with previous events; or the new events may interrupt preceding currents by resetting all or a significant number of components that have gone before, without regard for their values in current event clusters. Pressing suggests that the choice between association or interruption depends on the player's tolerance level for repetition – and in music therapy, as suggested, the choice would also depend on therapeutic demands.

Finally, in clinical improvisation we cannot think simply in terms of musical intention and actual form. Another dimension generates, and is generated by, the music, and this is the personal and interpersonal one. We can see the global event as something like that depicted in Figure 6.2.

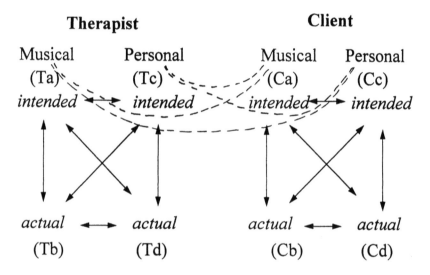

Figure 6.2 The intended and actual forms, and the personal and interpersonal dimensions, in clinical improvisation

We can see the improvisation as a four-point shifting event: thus (Tc) T's personal/clinical intention (e.g. to contain and meet C's distress and agitation), is formed from what T receives of C's musical utterances (Cb) (e.g. C's taut, unsteady rhythmic clusters). In order to actualise her clinical/interpersonal intentions, T has to form a musical intention (Ta) (e.g. T makes musical decisions about timbre, tempo, melody and rhythm), which then needs to be translated into (Tb) (T's improvisation meets C's rhythmic patterns). The client receives Tb and, as a result, forms a personal intention (Cc), which they translate into a musical intention (Ca), which is actualised (Cb) for the therapist to receive. And so on.

Creating and Conveying Musical Structure

We cannot leave this discussion on music cognition without a word about musical structure. What is becoming evident, in all the above concepts, is that when we listen to music, we perceive *not* an arbitrary sequence of sounds but hierarchical levels of rhythmic and melodic units. Eric Clarke (1988) alerts us to two distinct psychological orientations in the performance of music, whether pre-composed or improvised. One aspect is that the musical structure is represented in a form that inputs our motor system, so that we perform the musical structure we have in mind; and another aspect is that the expressive features of a musical performance draw attention to, and convey an understanding of, a particular interpretation of the piece's musical structure.

We saw earlier Cook's (1990) distinction between 'musical' and 'musicological' listening. Musical listening, he suggests, is 'listening for pleasure', providing listeners with an opportunity to lose themselves in the music. This quality of musical listening allows access to another reality, and this reality is non-dualistic, in that our consciousness, while listening, is 'other' – and separate from the reality of the external world. Musicological listening, on the other hand, refers to any type of listening whose purpose, rather than being direct gratification, is to establish facts about the music, to confirm aspects of style, structure or a technical aspect of its performance, and to formulate theories about it.

Bearing both Cook's and Clarke's distinctions in mind, how, might we ask, do music therapists listen? Do we listen in either the musical or musicological mode, or both, or another way altogether? Do we think in terms of therapists listening through various screens: musical, musicological, personal, interpersonal – all of which make up the whole listening experience? For the time being, let us concentrate on musical listening and structuring.

Psychologists Robert West, Peter Howell and Ian Cross (1991) remind us that a defining feature of music is that it is structured, so that in improvising music we are generating structure as we go along. This structure, being generated in our minds, inputs into our motor functioning, which realises the mental structuring through sounds. At the same time, however, music therapists need to ensure that in joint music improvisations, they and the client share an understanding of the musical structure – even if their understanding is not at the same cognitive level.

But what *is* structure, ask West *et al.*? Is it a relational concept, a way of relating various bits to one another; is it the decomposing of a piece of music into its interrelated sub-units, (rather like a hierarchy made up of small parts, grouped together to form larger and larger groups, like the tree structure in Schenkerian musical analysis)? Or rather, is musical structure an 'attribute' in the sense that it is something essential and characteristic that can be found among different pieces of music? Cook (1990) asks whether structure is the way that we 'perceive' musical movement, i.e., make sense of it. He asks whether understanding musical structure enhances the aesthetic experience of listening to music – in other words, is it necessary to understand the structure for the music to be meaningful? Although his own view is that perceptual acts are not essential to aesthetic pleasure, Cook reminds us of Schenker's view: that musical structure demonstrates, not so much how people actually perceive music when they listen, but rather how music ought to be heard if the composer's full and complex intentions are to be absorbed.

In considering structure in the hierarchical sense (as we might do when applying Schenkerian analysis to a piece of music), then a question emerges regarding how music therapists listen to the recording of music therapy improvisations after the sessions. When, for instance, do music therapists choose to listen to higher level structures; when do we listen to the smaller units? What is it that triggers a shift in the hierarchical level that is being focused on? Does the level of listening depend on the extent of therapeutic/interpersonal significance of the excerpt? Is the trigger connected to our memory of the actual session, that 'something happened'? Is it related to a variation in style, e.g. a move towards inconsistent or 'ungrammatical' music? Sandra Brown's (1992) metaphor of a map having different 'degrees of magnification' parallels the idea of listening at different hierarchical structural levels. She suggests that one kind of 'listening map' might 'zoom in' on the micro-musical event: what happened between this note and that, how was this rhythmic motif developed? A larger-scale listening map might have a wider angle: what is the overall structure of this piece – is it binary, is it a 'theme and variation', a rondo form, and so on – what Clarke (1990) calls the unified conception, that takes in the entire improvisation at a single glance, as he puts it (Figure 6.3)? Here the listener is able to hear the piece as a unity, from the highest level (a) down to the lowest level (b) where each note is represented. Other kinds of maps would listen from the interactive perspective, and others from the interpersonal – but this is not our concern right now.

(a) higher level of
    musical structure

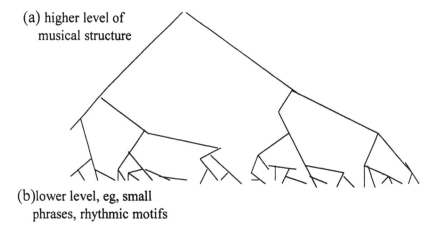

(b) lower level, eg, small
    phrases, rhythmic motifs

Figure 6.3 Global listening – the listener is able to take in all levels of a piece's structure

From a music therapy perspective, we might use Schenker's hierarchical 'tree' model of musical structure, that links smaller units at lower levels to form higher order units, to explain the shift in awareness from lower order to increasingly complex and global musical processes in a series of sessions. Most music therapists are familiar with having to focus on a simple and small rhythmic pattern as an initial step of 'coming together' with a client. Cognitively speaking, this could be a lower level structural unit. As the client is increasingly able to meet and respond to the lower level pattern in a sustained manner, the music therapist might then extend the improvisation into a longer phrase, thus linking together smaller units and moving to a higher order of musical structure.

For example, in their case study of Logan, Paul Nordoff and Clive Robbins (1977) take Logan through the musical steps culminating in a triumphant march entitled, 'Here is a Boy', that links together the shorter units. We can explain this process by suggesting that the therapists generate higher order structure levels for the child to develop towards – finally reaching a (triumphant) stage where the structural and 'learnt' aspects of the sessions can be transcended into sheer exuberance and excitement of the song and all that it has come to mean for the therapists and for Logan. The boy is first taken through steps of assimilating the lower order units until they become imprinted, so to speak, as musical schematas, and he can absorb these and reproduce them 'automatically', while concentrating on higher level units such as phrasing, and then higher expressive features which convey a thorough grasp of the march's structure.

Eric Clarke[1] provides a helpful model in describing how musical structure is developed in the course of a music improvisation. He suggests that in jazz, for instance, the first event (M1) may be worked out in advance or developed through the improvisation. The relationship between M1 and the subsequent collection of events can be organised in different ways, and he proposes three principles. In the first (Figure 6.4), the hierarchical structure is worked out to some extent. In the second (Figure 6.5), the principle of a chain operates, where each musical event is triggered by the previous ones. In the third possibility (Figure 6.6), the improviser has a range of event repertoires, and these events are selected in random order and made to relate to one another.

When therapist and client are together generating a single musical structure, each partner needs to communicate to the other their own understanding of the musical structure since, as Clarke points out, any piece of music is open to more than one structural interpretation. Clarke suggests that solo performers form an understanding of the musical structure, or decide between structural alternatives, and limit the extent of the piece's ambiguity in a stable manner. The role of musical expression, he says, is to project a particular meaning for a given musical structure. One way of achieving this is to emphasise the Gestalt properties already evident in the structure, or, where the music is structurally neutral, to establish the Gestalt features. For example, changes in dynamic articulation or timing gradients, or the subtle modification of accent, creates and indicates boundaries in the music's grouping structures.

The generating and conveying of musical structure in music therapy improvisation is compounded by the therapeutic dimension of the improvisation. Any of Clarke's three structural principles might, at any point, be dismissed in the interests of the patient's personal needs. However, where the therapeutic demands are precisely that therapist and client together experience a structured improvisation, with the principles of personal coherence, co-operation and organisation that these invite from the person, then, as in Logan's case, the therapist needs to ensure that each event is assimilated by the client before the next sequence is introduced. Here, it would seem, there is no room for structural ambiguity. However, it would appear that the greater the degree of interpersonal trust and intimacy between therapist and client, then the more room there is for a high degree of ambiguity in the generating of structure. Indeed the most exciting and inspiring moments in

---

1 Figures 6.4–6.6 draw direct inspiration from Eric Clarke's figures. However, here they are somewhat simplified, in keeping with the emphasis and bias of this discussion.

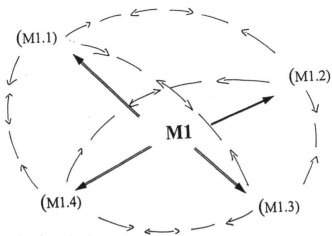

Figure 6.4 The relationship between a pre-set musical idea (M1) and improvisational ideas triggered from it

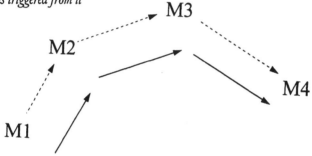

Figure 6.5 The relationship between ongoing musical events (⟶) and temporally preceding ones (←−−)

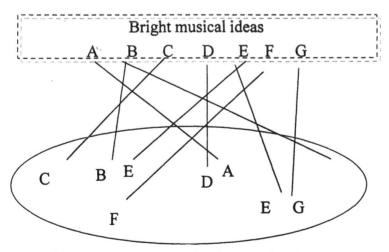

Figure 6.6 The improvisations contains and combines a number of musical ideas, all of which pre-exist, in the players' musical repertoire

spontaneous music therapy improvisation (which may be considered akin to free jazz improvisation at this level), are when neither the therapist nor the client is certain of the other's mental modelling of the improvisation as it unfolds, but, as though by supernatural synchronicity, both arrive at a cadential moment which suddenly clicks the preceding ambiguities into place. My experience is that such moments are often followed by a burst of excitement, manifested in laughter, an intense vocal sound or a highly charged silence.

Musical Style

Finally, I want to address, very briefly, the place of musical style in music therapy improvisation, since, as we saw earlier, music therapists may choose to develop an improvisation along the rules of a particular style. Mary Louise Serafine (1988) alerts us to the fact that musical styles continuously change, evolving over time into new styles and then becoming obsolete. A symptom of style change is the incessant writing of new music.

It is worth clarifying the distinction between 'style' and 'idiom'. Idiom may be thought of as a basic, coherent unit which may be a melodic fragment, rhythmic patterns, a tonal scale or a harmonic idiom which is transferable across musical styles. Thus, as Hargreaves (1986) points out, whereas Beethoven and the Beatles might use similar harmonic idioms, they cannot be said to belong to the same musical style.

Musical style refers to a body of compositions that share similar features: the composers, listeners and performers recognise these special features as being characteristic of a particular style, such as jazz, folk, rock, baroque, and so on. Serafine suggests that style change results from the interaction between members of a musical community, i.e., composers, performers and listeners. True style, she says, is a cultural matter, and is never invented in isolation from some audience, no matter how small – much in the way that a group shares an evolving language or system of discourse.

Serafine's statements about style changes relate beautifully to music therapy improvisation: the session may be seen as a social or cultural microcosm, in which therapist and client are, together, the composers, performers and audience. Together they create improvisations in certain musical styles. During the course of ongoing therapy sessions, this micro-musical community may pass through different stylistic genres (not in a chronological, historical sense) as a result of therapeutic demands. For example, during three years of working with a boy who had cognitive learning deficits, we created, explored and journeyed through marches of the Souza persuasion, Scottish folk, Negro spiritual and our own version of romantic schmaltz. Each of these stylistic genres waxed and waned at different periods of our work, some to reappear later, while some styles were explored concurrently. There seemed to be a natural, rather than forced, time for these stylistic genres to emerge and to disappear.

According to Sundberg and Lindstrom (1991), knowing a musical style enables us to hear and to generate what is appropriate and possible in an improvisation, in terms of sequence of pitches, duration, chords, and so on. They call this stylistic coherence in a piece of music 'grammatical'. Our minds can imagine the structure and the style that we generate in the act of improvisation, and we know when we depart from the style – i.e. when we move to ungrammatical music.

As improvising music therapists we create music with clients from our 'learnt' repertoire of musical styles. In other words, we are familiar with the attributes or idiomatic characteristics that make up a musical style – and this is an aspect of learning clinical improvisation techniques – although, as we have seen, the purpose of clinical improvisation is not to generate a particular musical style or musical structure. In the course of forming a therapeutic, clinical relationship with the client, the musical medium has its own power and colour which, as proficient musicians, music therapists naturally draw on in the course of this therapeutic/musical relating, in the same way that psychotherapists might use idiomatic language or the particular connotation of a phrase – or even of a folk tale or of a poem – in order to capture something about the therapeutic relationship.

Music therapy improvisation is peculiar in the sense that the (musically versed) therapist and the (musically unversed or less versed) client, together seem to arrive at a particular musical style. How does this happen? As with much of our preceding discussion, how can the music therapist be sure that she is not imposing/colonising the client's playing with what she, the therapist, has in her (musical) mind? We need to remind ourselves that clinical improvisation is a joint event: not a matter of the therapist listening to the client playing, but the two of them are in the music together: together they generate, interpret and extend the music. In this context, the therapist remains highly sensitive, alert and responsive to rhythmic, dynamic, melodic or harmonic cues from the client, who is unaware (and uncognisant) of musical style *per se*.

As we saw earlier, the client's awareness may well be at a basic level of generating basic perceptual grouping mechanisms and organising patterns at a simple level – which does not mean that this is musically uninteresting. Far from it: we saw earlier that the Gestalt principles of symmetry, regularity and proximity are fundamental to the human experience of music, and, indeed, Lerdahl (1991) suggests that we organise experience into structured categories: when music becomes too fragmented and inaccessible, we organise experience into schemata which provide stable reference points, helping us to make sense of the music. The client's cues act as a musical 'trigger' for the therapist, who then weaves the client's offerings, creating and developing a musical style that is the most appropriate and the most congruent with the client's playing. It is the therapist's task to ensure that this musical style generates shared meaning between the players. The meaning may be different for each of the players, in the sense that different aspects may 'mean' different things for each person, but their meaning must be attached to the musical experience that happens between them, and that both players create.

In Conclusion

These models of the active cognitive framework relate directly to music therapy improvisation techniques, in that they provide music therapists with a vocabulary for describing the tools and musical processes of their craft, even if they do not describe the inter-personal psychological/dynamic processes that are generated and elicited through the music between the therapist and client. Clinical improvisation is more than two people improvising music together, but in order to create this 'more than', music therapists first learn to construct and develop mental/musical schemata, construct and unravel musical styles, become familiar with improvisational techniques and their mechanisms. During this learning they begin to detach these from conventionally coded musical vocabulary, so that the musical constructs are heard and conceptualised, not only as music but as potentially eliciting, inviting and developing a personal relationship through the improvisation.

For example, instead of hearing and playing a tango as part of a Latin American idiom, we might need to use such a motif in clinical improvisation in a psychological way. In work with the Scots client described earlier – a man whose severe alcohol dependency was complicated with physically abusive acts towards his family – I heard a tight, driven, quasi-militaristic beat on the snare drum. This tightness can be conceptualised musically as well as personally and interpersonally. There was no breath, breadth or respite in his rapid beating, and this, together with his deafening noise level, made my attempts to meet him, improvising from the piano, rather feeble. I could match neither his prodigious energy nor his monumental dynamic level. Psychologically I knew that unless I was able to meet him through the music, as a result of my psychological understanding, the potential for a therapeutic relationship would remain severely limited. Musically this psychological insight translated into the tango rhythm, and it was this that 'got' him: when played strongly, with an exaggerated accent on the second beat, the syncopated crotchet note could also be played/interpreted as being a quaver followed by a rest, as shown in Figure 6.7.

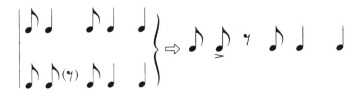

Figure 6.7 Tango (1)

This 'rest' caught his imagination – and this prompted ambiguity in the music: the rest enabled a movement towards a new cognitive schema, through the combination/addition of a new feature. Thus he was able to check his rapid beating for a split second, introducing a 'lift', and this narrow and tight lift in his playing began to widen almost imperceptibly. The tango rhythm then became increasingly ambiguous, and our music-making floated, so to speak, between a conventional tango motif and, by shifting the accent (and thereby the metre), we explored, spontaneously and with split-second shifts of emphasis, various 'ways of being' in our joint music-making (see Figure 6.8).

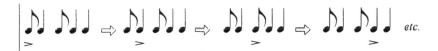

Figure 6.8 Tango (2)

It is insufficient and incomplete to describe this event only in terms of schemata, time referents, style, idiom, musical structure, and so on, although we could quite easily do so. We undoubtedly make use of cognitive and perceptual processes: for example, in order to gain an impression of this patient's rapid playing, my musical perception was activated; I then interpreted his beating according to my mental schema, and my musical imagination enabled the schema to 'attach' itself to a tango motif, already present in my musical vocabulary. This motif generated harmonic textures that feature in the Latin American idiom, and this in turn provided a musical vocabulary for melodic contours. This musical style seemed psychologically appropriate for the quality of this client's machismo, and also appropriate for the quality of our interaction.

In introducing the tango motif at the piano, my capacity to actualise my musical intention in the improvisation was activated, and the patient was able to reproduce this motif, thereby showing his perceptual and neurological intactness. He too was able to perceive, to 'intend' and to 'actualise'. We could say that the accents of the tango provided an invariant, which attached us both to the same music. We could both recognise the invariant and depend upon its predictability. The predictable musical phrase that emerged over the tango rhythm provided a time referent – we both came to know the sections of our improvisation. I then introduced ambiguity in the rhythmical/metrical structure by shifting the metre and accent of the tango: this caused us both to 'reconstruct' a new invariant, until the next structural shift. It was, perhaps, this very ambiguity that allowed the client to enter into a joint musical event – he was able to make his own sense of the improvisation, and by contributing responsively, albeit from his own cognitive perspective, he gave me further cues, which then caused me to revise my playing. There was a musical – and a psychological – 'fit' between us.

None of this description would be sufficient to describe the total therapeutic event, just as none of this would capture the magic of a jazz improvisation in which two players inter-cue each other, sparking off musical ideas. These models and descriptions fall short of addressing the therapeutic event, the personal, intimate, inter-engagement between therapist and client – but this is no reason to ignore them. Indeed we might say that by describing only the therapeutic, the interpersonal and the psychological, our description is as limited. It is, after all, the musical act which is the emotional act.

Colin Lee (1989) has already made this point. His meticulous description and analysis of complex improvisations with clients suffering from HIV/AIDS, uses a Schenkerian model of musical analysis, showing the hierarchical structural levels of the improvisations. This analysis does not convey the inter-personal, the therapeutic event, but it goes a long way to explaining how it is that two people's playing interweaves so intimately in music therapy improvisation.

Finally, a perspective from cognitive music psychology provides insights into improvisatory mechanisms and, more pressing perhaps, provides frameworks and models through which we can engage with enriching dialogues with music psychologists and music theorists. To return to Sandra Brown's 'degrees of magnification' (1992), each of the various levels of looking at the music therapy session has its own limitations: just as a micro-detailed exploration of the musical events restricts the overall 'aerial' view, so the unified global view lacks details unless we are truly able to conceptualise all levels at once which, as Clarke suggests, is rather an ideal. By gaining an understanding of perceptual mechanisms and theoretical modellings of how we listen and how we understand music, music therapists can choose from a wider palette for describing their practice, not just from a position of being 'similar to' other arts therapies, but of knowing how to explain what it is that distinguishes music therapy from music.

PART II

CHAPTER 7

Meaning in Relationship
The Music Between

Colin entered the therapy room, holding his mother's hand. The room contained a snare drum...a cymbal...a pair of small beaters or drumsticks, a tambourine, two handchimes (on a wooden bench), and two small chairs, one larger chair, an upright piano and piano stool.

On seeing me, Colin threw himself onto the floor, where he lay prone and motionless. I remained where I was, by the bench. I tentatively tapped a few beats on the tambourine and paused. Colin showed no response or reaction...I began to sing softly, while trying to gauge his mood, and immediately Colin screamed and 'drummed' his feet on the floor, his rage soon escalating to a full-scale temper tantrum. To meet the intensity and match of the tonal-rhythmic emotional characteristics of Colin's screaming and kicking, I began communicating with him from the piano, using intense, full-bodied and sometimes dissonant harmonies in a minor key. This seemed to resonate with and acknowledge some of the emotional tension and pathos in his sounds. After repeating this twice and pausing for about the same phrase-length between playing, I noticed that Colin's screaming was not only in the tonality of the music, but was showing more clearly defined tonal-rhythmic elements of the music with which I had matched his initial sounds. His 'drumming' feet had begun to acquire an emotionally expressive organisation in the music.

(Robarts 1996, pp.150–51)

In reading Jacqueline Robarts' description of her work with this three-and-a-half-year-old autistic boy, it is clear that music therapy improvisation can generate a context which is not only intermusical, but inter-personal. Robarts sings, the child screams, drums his feet on the floor, and the therapist matches this intensity in her music. The music may not have sounded particularly 'nice' or particularly 'musical'. The participants in this improvisation – in this case Colin and Robarts – together create the improvisation. Although Colin does not have the musical know-how to improvise and, at this stage, could hardly be said to be improvising musically, he is, nevertheless, part of what the therapist is doing: she refers to him in creating a sound form that embodies both the quality of his acts and how she receives them. As the weekly sessions progress, the therapist continues to weave his acts, and his responses to her, as music, so that Colin and Robarts begin to experience themselves and one another directly and intimately through the jointly created, non-verbal sound form. This relating has many aspects to it: the nature of contact between therapist and child, the shifts between contact and non-contact, and the quality and aspects of the shifts themselves.

All, and any, of these give the therapist a picture of the child. This picture, however, needs to make sense. How does the therapist know that what Colin does is significant? That it is not 'just' a musical game? That the context is inter-personal as well as intermusical? That the surface acts – the sounds – mean more than just the sounds themselves? How is the link made between the personal and the musical? Moreover, just to complicate the picture, how does the music therapy improvisation fit with his autism – how does the therapist report on the work to her colleagues?

Music Therapy and Illness

Music therapy may not directly address the client's complaint, which may be severe headaches, depression, a neurological problem, a communication deficit, a mental/physical/neurologically based disability or, like Colin, autism. Music therapy improvisation appeals not only to the symptoms but to the whole person, including those aspects that are not 'ill', and including those aspects of the client that have only an obtuse relationship to 'the illness'. David Aldridge (1993a) reminds us that music therapy cannot restrict itself to the medical axis of health–illness. In music therapy, 'ill-health' becomes meaningful in a new way, and music therapy becomes an experience which does not necessarily point directly towards 'the illness'. Colin's music therapy experience was one of increasing emotional contact between him and the music therapist, and the context for this contact was not just his autism, it was the whole of himself. The creative arts potentiate us: they elicit the tension between who we are and how we might be, and in music therapy this happens in an interpersonal context. Within this context, to think of clients as 'improving' or as music therapy 'working' is limited ground, although appealing, in that these well-established concepts form part of global and dominant models of illness/health – and 'treatment'.

Perhaps rather than fitting in with pre-existing models, we might think of complementing them. Many music therapists work as part of multidisciplinary teams, where meaning needs to be negotiated between all members of the team. My own experience of being part of a multidisciplinary team in an adult psychiatric hospital, was that through music therapy I gained an immediate and penetrating sense of the client, often within the first minutes of the clinical improvisation. I 'knew' why aspects of the sessions were significant – this was not a musical-intuitive knowing, but a clinically informed intuitive knowing, based on the direct musical experience with the client. However, my attempts at conveying this 'knowing' to the team were, initially, frustrating for us all. I grappled to speak a language that was not exclusively couched in musical terms, and yet to speak 'metaphorically' did not feel quite right either. I often felt de-skilled and ineffectual at team meetings. Over several months of working together, the multidisciplinary team learnt my idiosyncratic, music therapy language, and at the same time I learnt their learning of my language. Gradually we all grasped the highly relevant – and not always tangible – contribution of music therapy to the ward rounds. There was no simple assessment system whereby I could position the patient on a scale from 1 to 10, and in any case, even had there been one, it might have prevented us (and absolved us) from intuitively grasping, as a team, the complexities of the patient.

How might we frame the music therapy experience? We might look at Colin through various lenses, as we looked at Xolile at the beginning of this book. The example with Colin, however, highlights the fact that he and the therapist could not converse, through words, in the sense that Xolile and I could had we wanted to and, indeed, at times, did. And yet, as one follows Robarts' description, it is clear that she got to 'know' this child and he her: it is the very mechanisms of this 'knowing' that are addressed in the next two chapters.

It is clear that it was not Colin's 'musicality' that enabled him to orientate and respond to the therapist's sound forms. Somehow he recognised that these sound forms had something to do with him: something fundamental and simple – almost natural. How Colin made that connection between himself and the sounds is the focus of this section on music in non-verbal communication. It is, of course, limiting to think of music therapy only as non-verbal communication. Music therapy is much more than that.

These explorations do not propose that music therapy practice 'parallels' non-verbal communication. Rather a case is made for the therapeutic power of clinical improvisation. Do we really understand how and why music 'works' in music therapy? Why music is inherently therapeutic? Quite apart from the hope that some concepts from this literature explain and describe music therapy improvisation, they can also usefully be drawn into the way that music therapists think about – and explain – their work. Had I had these concepts in mind at the team meetings, my practice itself might not have altered but I would have had access to a broader language, and to concepts, with which to describe these events.

Being Humanly Conscious

In exploring the literature on non-verbal communication, I experienced some scepticism as to why these musical mechanisms were particularly *human* phenomena. In noting the various features of non-verbal communication, it seemed that many of these features could be applied as effectively to the higher echelons of the animal world, which, for the most part, do not speak and yet which 'know' each other. Before bringing this literature towards the realm of music therapy (which is, after all, practised primarily with human beings), it seems important to clarify what makes us humanly conscious.

All living beings – human and non-human – respond to, and impinge on, the environment with different degrees of sensitivity and effectiveness. Somewhere along the spectrum, sensitivity and impingement include a dimension of consciousness of self within them. This dimension brings with it an awareness of our environment, self-consciousness about our presence in the environment and a capacity for sharing meaning. These degrees of sensitivity and responsiveness may be portrayed in music therapy improvisation: here, rather than being a feature of lower plant life, non-responsiveness or very limited responsiveness may be read as a feature of the relationship between therapist and client.

Nicholas Humphrey (1992) has outlined the range of these sensitivities or susceptibilities. At one end of the range, the 'locally reactive sensitivity', a living organism responds locally, directly and uncomplicatedly to a surface stimulus (e.g., the skin of a horse reacting to a fly): in terms of clinical improvisation, we might think of the lower levels of Nordoff and Robbins' (1977) musical communicativeness scale, where the child/client experiences the music peripherally, where their response to the therapist is 'evoked', reflexive, almost a 'knee-jerk reaction to a change, without this reaction necessarily being at a level of expressiveness of 'self'. At a higher level are organisms that can discriminate between, and respond differently to, different kinds of stimuli (i.e., that have a range of reactions which relate to the nature of the stimulus). At a higher level of Nordoff and Robbins' scale is the child who senses a distinction between one musical stimulus and another: the child's responses are 'musically directed', and this response adapts to the particular musical stimulus, rather than simply 'responding' in any way or in a limited way, to the stimulus. Next on Humphrey's range are organisms, at a higher level, that give value to stimuli, responding to them as good or bad, as significant or insignificant: in music therapy the child may be responding to music, and affecting the music in an intentional way, motivated by feelings of pleasure or displeasure. At a higher level still, organisms have the mental capacity to be sensitive to the 'action patterns', or representations of stimuli, and to respond to these rather than to the 'external' or 'surface structure' of stimuli. This is moving towards a reciprocity of mental life, in the sense that the living being can imagine the essence of the stimulus and respond according to this imagination. At the highest extreme of sensitivity, there is a complex and sophisticated response to a stimulus, which we respond to, and interpret as, a sign of something else, as in our coding and decoding intention and meaning through our use of language. In music therapy, at this level, the improvising partners share meaning through the improvisation: the improvisation is not just about itself but about more than itself: it portrays meaning that is personal, complex and shareable with another.

When I watch our old ginger cat being disturbed and challenged by our lively 11-month-old male kitten, I see aspects of these sensitivities in motion. The two animals orientate towards one another, move in synchrony with one another, the younger cat displays forceful whacks, dives, bites and rolls, while the older cat's movements are a co-responding dance. I also note the old ginger cat's inability to counteract in a quick enough tempo, coming off worse and spitting, and, as a consequence his dominance in social rank within the household is being challenged. All of these movements and correspondences involve signals that are neurologically based, and that are shared among the species. They also involve musical elements. These are displayed not only in the tempo, intensity, rhythm and phrasing of the movements and yowls, but also in the crescendo and diminuendo, in the accellerando and diminuendo of the animals' energy and aggression. But do these animals have a consciousness about themselves in relation to one another that is *beyond* their singular experience? Beyond what Vygotsky (1986) terms 'lower' natural mental functions such as elementary perceptions, memory, attention and will? Does their consciousness take into account a 'cat culture' that they share with other members of the species? Is there a cat-lore, are there legends of past heroic cats, victorious cats, cat philosophers that get passed on to new generations? I somehow think not.

What is it that makes us distinctly human? How do we acquire the imagination to act responsively and coherently in the world, and see the world, not as the sum of movements coloured by tensions and resolutions, but as a conveyer, and receiver, of complex and multi-faceted abstract and concrete concepts and meanings? How do we, as human beings, do more than just react to what another does, rather than reacting to the *meaning* of the other's acts? How do we become part of the human culture; how do we get to co-respond with our human world, rather than remain excluded, bewildered and socially unconscious? Where and how do we connect the musical elements that seem to exist in all biological beings that pulsate, move, expand and contract, with that exclusively human capacity to generate, share and exchange meaning that is personal, social and cultural?

It seems to me that these questions are at the heart of understanding and describing music therapy. Colin and the therapist were not just gravitating towards one another's acts, in the way of the two cats. The depth and multi-faceted aspects of 'meanings' assigned to the acts, by the therapist at first, enabled her to 'know' Colin: to 'know' what was going on inside him, and how to respond to this. Was Colin passively receiving the therapist's sound forms? Were his acts coincidentally, reflexively related to the therapist, or was the coincidence created within her mind? And in any case, how could she 'know' what this child was feeling?

The next chapters will help to clarify why it is that music is so much part of our lives, as human beings – not just because our heartbeats may speed up or slow down, be regular or irregular, or because our speaking voices may be sing-song in character, staccato or legato, or sforzando or diminuendo. All of these, of course, are musical concepts. But this is not the whole picture. By visiting the literature on non-verbal communication, I hope to clarify how it is that Colin and his therapist came to 'know' each other – and how I might have been better able to describe my work in multidisciplinary team meetings.

CHAPTER 8

Songs without Words
Music in Communication[1]

In this chapter I focus almost exclusively on those aspects of non-verbal communication that are relevant to clinical improvisation, before drawing these into music therapy. In order to explore the personal/musical mechanisms of music therapy improvisation, I begin with a description of musical features of non-verbal communication between human beings, since it seems that it is these very features that are elicited in clinical improvisation, through a medium that is particularly suited to portraying them. After looking at the musical features of non-verbal communication, I turn the looking glass the other way, so to speak, to look at the (non-verbal) communicative features of clinical improvisation in music therapy.

All over the world, human beings communicate through language: we symbolically attach words to events, objects and concepts, and it is through words that we share the meaning of events, concepts and objects with one another. However, despite the universal presence, and ongoing evolution, of complex language-based rules and culturally coded symbols, words alone do not suffice. Words are accompanied by gestures, are coloured by intensity of tempo, vocal texture, by facial expressions, and so on. Human beings everywhere 'tune into' not just the words that are being said. Moreover, anyone who has found themselves in a foreign-language culture, has had the experience of being able to 'get the feel of' another person, without being able to speak their language. Mothers and new-born infants have no words: they communicate intimately and directly with one another – and know one another.

Even as adults, it seems that a significant aspect of our experience of ourselves, of one another, of the world and of ourselves in the world, does

---

1   I am especially grateful to Jackie Robarts for her input on this, and the following, chapter.

not fit exclusively within verbal thought and language. Rather these other significant aspects of ourselves, and of our experience, exist somewhere alongside our verbal selves, complement them, indeed are part of them, and can bypass words altogether if and when necessary. This is not to say, of course, that we can function without verbal processes – but at the same time, our intellectually insistent Western culture places a particular emphasis on verbal thought and language – which, of course, all too aptly accompanies – and dictates – the mechanistic model of illness and health. In considering how we communicate in music therapy, I want to focus on those aspects of our humanity and of human consciousness that do not fit into words, since it is our essential 'being' that is captured by music therapy improvisation. How do we begin to formulate this? Certain aspects of the literature on non-verbal communication have elicited some critical concepts that help to clarify, to explain music therapy improvisation, and I now turn to this literature for the rest of this chapter – while not pretending to offer an overview of this fascinating field.

Communicating Comes Naturally

What has become clear, in the last 20 years of research into infant development, is that being part of the human condition is a highly sophisticated and complex experience that is ready to be activated from birth. We are ready to know the world without words. Trevarthen and Aitken (1994) suggest that the psychological/physiological mechanisms that pattern the embryo and foetal brain, constrain and direct the infant's brain, after birth, in exploring, in being attentive, in not only looking for care and protection, but in being part of the pleasurable and unpleasurable effects of communication with their caregivers. This effective and direct communication with another human being, usually the mother or primary caregiver, colours the way that the infant gets to know the world. The emotional quality of this first relationship has critical implications for the infant's cognitive growth.

John Bowlby (1969) talks about 'patterns of interaction' between mother and infant, that may be highly stable, and a source of satisfaction to each of the partners, in contrast to less stable and unsatisfactory patterns, which may result in ongoing personal lack of satisfaction and instability, separate from the mother–infant dyad. My frustration in team meetings, described in the previous chapter, was only assuaged when we – the team and I – could develop a more consistent and stable pattern of sharing and exchanging concepts. The initial music therapy interaction between Robarts and Colin (described earlier) can be described as 'incipient patterning'. But how did the therapist know that this approach would work, would 'meet' the child? Why did she not console the child with a soothing lullaby, instead?

Mothers and new-born infants know each other intimately and have a direct emotional experience of one another, despite the infant's lack of access to culturally shared signals and, more especially, to language. (Colin might have not made sense of the soothing lullaby – despite its cultural connotations. And, in any case, he reacted adversely to the voices of strangers.) These studies clarify, and help to conceptualise, how this direct, non-verbal communication is possible. They have challenged the dominance of those psychological theories that propose that we are born with uncoordinated minds (as in William James' idea of the booming buzz of the baby's world) that respond reflexively with or through physiologically based responses; and that our development and functioning are dependent upon highly rational cognition of the world: i.e., the 'active' child gathering information from the 'passive' world. This literature also challenges the assumptions and inferences made about our inner, private experience, purely on the basis of observing and evaluating public behaviour – the domain of behavioural psychology. Thus the therapist did not assume or infer how Colin felt – she came to 'know' him directly.

Our innate capacity to seek optimal inter-personal relating, even as young infants, needs to be understood as part of our 'interpersonal intelligence' that is enormously flexible and co-ordinated. This interpersonal awareness, present from birth, enables us to experience the world not passively, but as agents in it, who receive from, and impinge on, the world in a co-ordinated, highly flexible manner. What is exciting for music therapists is that the nature of this capacity to engage with the world has a musical basis. Music is part of every infant's living experience of the world, not in the sense of hearing nursery rhymes or lullabies, but in the presence of the musical (and unintegrated) elements of rhythm, tempo, intensity, contours, patterning, and so on. When Colin raged, kicked and screamed, the therapist was able to decode the 'musical' information – the quality – of his acts, and share this information with him, in this way becoming part of his emotional life.

It seems to me that we need to understand this musical basis of our early life thoroughly, since it makes a crucial link between (1) the oft-cited presence of (disparate) musical elements in our physiology and neurology, and (2) our understanding of how and why music is an effective therapeutic medium. In other words, since the elements of music are essential to our earliest – and natural – interactions and impressions, although not in the conventions of our culture – it seems appropriate that music – even when culturally coded – continues to have such powerful resonances for us in our adult lives. The extension of this power is the use of music by therapist and client, in order to communicate with one another, and rekindle the primacy of the powerfully non-verbal, and pre-verbal, ways of being.

Let us leave Colin's music therapy aside, and attempt to clarify the relevance of this literature for music therapy improvisation.

Mothers and Infants

Psychologists who have observed the interplay of feelings between mother and alert new-born attest to the innateness of both the mother's and baby's susceptibility to one another's feelings and communicative acts. Infants do not 'learn' how to feel or how to communicate feelings (Beebe 1982; Beebe *et al.* 1985; Trevarthen 1993). Both Trevarthen (1979, 1987) and Stern (1985) state that the infant is born with the motivation to engage in an intimate emotional relationship from birth. Not only must the infant and mother 'know' one another since, biologically, the infant is utterly dependent on the mother for the fulfilment of physical needs, but the mother too needs to 'know' the baby's needs. They both need to share meaning: to have a common experience of themselves and one another, so that the infant may experience itself within the context of a relationship. Quite aside from its role in fulfilling the infant's physical needs, this intimate emotional relationship is critical for the infant in developing a sense of him or herself as a social being and part of a human community.

The primitive state of the infant's mind is ready to be aware, is actively present to other persons and is receptive to, and communicative with, others. Far from being mentally incoherent or only reflexively responsive, infants are highly motivated and make efforts to engage with the world. This innate motivation persists, despite the infant existing outside the social culture of the persons around them – and also, of course, despite the absence of language. The infant's capabilities for social communication are coherent: the infant communicates cohesively and sensitively with others, from a very early age (Murray and Trevarthen 1985, 1986). This confirms the opinions of the neuropsychologists Botez *et al.* (1983), who suggested that our brains have the capacity to detect patterns and to reproduce them. Thus there is an anatomical-physiological predisposition for our capacity to co-ordinate. This basic integrity enables the infant to hold together all behaviours and perceptions at a given moment, rather than experiencing others or the world as a disparate set of elements – the baby does not experience the flick of a hand, the smell of mother's body, the temperature of her body, the intensity of her voice, as separate and disconnected, but rather co-ordinates them as part of its global experience of being alive.

Babies and their mothers exchange information about themselves and about one another across modalities (Trevarthen 1986). In other words, the baby's feeling state is conveyed through facial expression, movement and vocal sound – the intensity, shape and motion of which present the baby as a co-ordinated being. This means that the intensity of the vocal sound corresponds with the intensity of the movement and of the facial grimace. The message, whether it is one of a state of calmness, urgency or lethargy, can be transferred across modes of expression, whether vocal, gestural or through facial expression.

It is not only the baby's brain that does the perceiving. The infant is *part of* this perceptual experience. Humphrey (1992) draws attention to the false separation between 'sensations and perception'. Sensations are affect-laden: whatever we do has an affective component – and sensations are part of our mental representations of something happening here and now, not just 'over there', but as *part of* perceptual acts. Thus the affective aspect of how we perceive is part of, and colours, the perceptual process. Although using different discourses, this corresponds with both Trevarthen (1986) and Ulrich Neisser (1976), who argue that perception cannot be divorced from the (feeling) self in the act of perceiving. The psychological activity of perception generates an awareness and action of which the self – the emoting affective self – is an inherent part. In this case the infant is a curious, purposeful and effective seeker of information and regulator of movements who acts in focusing towards the object of interest. Unlike the cats, who seek to play/fight in a co-ordinated manner, the infant also has an awareness, as yet pre-verbal and unformed, of the self in relation to the other.

The quality of this seeking, receiving and engaging with the world can be conceptualised as a musical one. This 'music' is not just a feature of the mother–infant vocalisations, which might approach what we consider 'singing' – but rather it is a part of their total/global gestures, co-ordinated into a perceptual whole. However, Papousek and Papousek (1981, 1989, 1991), who have concentrated on mother–infant vocalisations in exploring this exchange and sharing of communication, make some arresting points. They suggest that parents respond to infants' earliest vocalisations as being *communicatively* meaningful, rather than as being 'musical', and this reinforces the infant's capacity to use his or her voice in a communicative sense – to anticipate a response from the other rather than vocalising into an interpersonal vacuum. The Papouseks' analysis of the prosodic aspects of mother–infant vocalisations reveal each partner's vocalisations taking into account the other partner's utterances. Each partner adapts the stresses and rhythmic features of their vocalisations interactionally: they are not uttered into a communicative void or a self-centred world, but rather take into account the quality of the other partner's utterances. The musical elements of infants' vocalisations do not develop as isolated or solitary phenomena, i.e. the 'musical' dimension of the vocalisation is not an aim in itself, and (most) parents do not vocalise with their infants in order to turn them into musicians. Rather the musical elements are part of the total behaviour within the intuitive and universal context of social interactions. Thus the linguistically sophisticated mother receives the communicative consciousness of her infant: she is aware of how the 'other' – the infant – receives her, and regulates her communicative acts to fit best with the infant's as yet non-linguistic mind.

Drawing from the Papouseks' earlier work, Mechthild Papousek (1996) suggests that parents and infants share a 'prelinguistic alphabet', or a code, that both infant-directed speech and infants' vocal sounds have in common. Both partners share salient features that enable them to reciprocate vocally with one another. This common code is supplemented by a social environment that corresponds, and complements, the infant's preferences and constraints, thus facilitating and supporting the infant's utterances. These early 'musical' interactions are not limited to vocal sounds, both occur through multi-modal patterns of communication that are complemented by the parent's multi-modal patterns of communicating.

The Papouseks' work has been substantiated by more recent analysis, which has shown that infants are predisposed to musical patterning (Unyk, Trehub, Trainor and Schellenberg 1992; Trehub, Unyk and Trainor 1993; Trehub and Trainor 1993), and that universal principles of auditory perception operate in infancy. Thus what Trehub calls 'prototypical' melodic and rhythmic groupings are not 'learnt' but are encoded in the infant's mind, apparently from birth. The processing of 'relational pitch' and 'temporal processing' seems to be a basic and uniquely human disposition, having to do with the nature of being human rather than with acquiring musical knowledge. Moreover, the infant's world is, as yet, uncluttered by words – the infant hears speech as contours and rhythm, and infant-directed speech is naturally sing-song in character, as though emphasising the prosodic, rather than the referential, meaning. Thus not only are infants sensitive and responsive to subtle shifts in their mothers' prosodic forms, especially shifts in intonation, rhythm and stress, but adults who are directing their speech towards infants modify their speech intuitively. Adults are not aware of their 'infant-directed' behaviour: they do not consciously set out to speak in a certain way when addressing infants. Infants, in turn, are extremely sensitive to the affective content of infant-directed adult speech. Trehub, Unyk and Trainor (1993b) show that infants contribute to maternal singing in that their presence affects the way that their mothers sing to them. This is in contrast with mothers singing the same song without the babies' presence: the babies' presence effected greater rhythmicity, a softer tone of voice, higher pitch and slower tempo. This seems to be intuitively based responsiveness, rather than a 'socially learnt' response to the mother.

The Papouseks (1989) suggest that expanded pitch range, frequent melodic repetition and continuous changes of pitch, as well as the prevalence of basic harmonic intervals, are features of what they call 'babytalk' or 'motherese', i.e. a language made up of specific prosodic features in order to engage the infant. Furthermore, the consistent presence of musical or prosodic elements in the mother's responses gives the infant a sense of predictability and familiarity – here we have the concept of stability and predictability being introduced to the infant within a communicative context at a very early age (Beebe et al. 1985; Papousek, Papousek and Bornstein 1985; Papousek, Papousek and Haekel 1987) – stability that is flexible and that makes for a satisfying pattern of 'attachment'.

Studies such as these, although clarifying different aspects of interactive features, have a common theme: they demonstrate the sensitivity and susceptibility of mother and infant to one another. It is not just the mother who adapts flexibly to her infant, but the infant, too, is alert, sensitive and responsive to the mother's own variations of communicative form. These capacities, it would seem, are innate rather than culturally learnt. Communicating comes naturally.

Self-Coherence (or: Do I Make Sense?)

For successful communication to occur between any two persons, not only must we receive our partner's communication as an integrated, unified whole, but in communicating we need to present ourselves coherently to the other person. We need to convey an integrated, organised whole being which is perceptually readable, rather than conveying a fragmented, disjointed set of behaviours.

The coherence of our actions, even as an infant, indicates the presence of an inner organisation of patterns and pulses which have their basis in the brain, thus enabling the physical and neurological co-activation of separate parts of the body (Trevarthen 1986). We do not 'learn' to be organised. Pribram (1982) states that the entire brain is involved in regulating behaviour: each part has a specific role in the totality of behaviour, thus ensuring smooth changes and stability of actions. An obvious exception is found in people who have a physical handicap as a result of, for example, cerebral palsy, brain injury or stroke. Their movements, speech, acts and gestures are distorted temporally, as they lack the control for smooth and fluid expressive and receptive functioning, which makes the meaning of their acts difficult to 'read'.

The famous and oft-cited work of psychologists Condon and Ogston (1966) demonstrates clearly the integration of various aspects of the self through detailed film analysis of two people speaking to one another. They show that various parts of the body move in a synchronised manner with the inflections of the speaker's voice, so that the speaker presents as an integrated, coherent, whole being. This intra-personal co-ordination they call 'self-synchrony', and contrast this normal communicative behaviour with that of schizophrenic patients, who lack variation of head movement, whose gaze is fixed rather than mobile and whose intonational contours are 'flat'. These schizophrenic patients show what the authors describe as 'self-dyssyn-chrony'. Bernieri and Rosenthal (1991) suggest that the co-ordination of body movements and speech is a fundamental skill that may facilitate the initial acquisition and development of language: the body may learn the physical manifestations and patterns of speech long before the infant is ready to speak. Moreover, synchrony has its own communicative function – not necessarily linked to speech – and may convey the degree of understanding, agreement or support that the listener is experiencing.

Colwyn Trevarthen calls this capacity for organising and co-ordinating states and processes within the self, 'subjectivity'. He writes that subjectivity is, '…the condition of being a co-ordinated subject, motivated to act with purpose in relation to the world outside' (Trevarthen 1980, p.324).

A sense of subjectivity – or an intra-subjective co-ordination – is crucial in interacting with the world. At the earliest time in our lives the sense of subjectivity is in our bodies: our senses receive the world through touch, smell, sound and vision, all of which are located within our bodies as infants, and this unified locus of reference is a foundation for expressing ourselves, receiving expression from, and co-ordinating and communicating with, another person.

Vitality Affects

One way of explaining what it is that 'holds us together' and enables us to experience the world and ourselves in it as a unified whole, is to use Daniel Stern's (1985) idea of 'vitality affects'. It seems that, from birth, the baby has a sense of self that is sustained during its evolving experience of the world. At first the baby's point of reference for linking together separate experiences is in the body, which the baby senses as a reference point with coherence, actions, feelings and the memory of all these. The baby forms relationships between isolated, disparate experiences through its reference point: thus the baby has the capacity to know that something that is seen, heard and touched may, in fact, be the same thing. In other words, the baby's experience of, say, a rattle, is that its sound, its touch and its colour belong to the same object and the same experience at that moment, rather than being three separate and disconnected experiences. The sound of the rattle is not separate from its form, nor is it separate from its weight, size or colour. The baby, says Stern, is able to make cross-modal transfers that enable it to recognise a correspondence between touch, smell, shape and sound, and this is the result of the innate design of the perceptual system, rather than being a product of repeated, learnt experiences, which is what the behavioural school of psychology would assert. More crucial, perhaps, is that babies have the capacity to correspond themselves to what they see and experience in the world. Stern draws from experiments which show three-week-old babies 'imitating' adults sticking out their tongues and opening their mouths, and proposes an innate correspondence between what the babies see and what they do. The tongue is experienced as belonging to the person sticking it out, and the baby recognises sufficient similarity between that person and itself for it to make a link between the other's acts and what it can do.

Thus infants appear to have an innate capacity for what Stern calls 'amodal perception'. This amodal form can be thought of as a property – such as shape, intensity level, motion, number and rhythm – that is experienced directly, and that can be 'lifted' off one person or thing and transferred across to another. Thus the infant can transfer something about the motion, intensity, the contour and shape of the tongue movement to its own attempts – quite apart from making the connection between where the tongue is situated in the body of the adult and the position of the tongue in its own body. This capacity for abstraction enables the infant to experience a world of perceptual unity. Babies perceive the amodal quality from any form of human expressive behaviour; they 'encode' this into what Stern suggests are 'still mysterious' amodal representations, and they can then recognise them in any of the sensory modes. The baby imitates adults sticking out their tongues by perceiving the quality of this movement: its shape, intensity and motion – which it then attempts to reproduce as one event. This attempt would be accompanied by body movements with the same amodal properties.

The term 'vitality affects' describes the amodal dynamic, kinetic quality of our experiences, and these impinge on our daily experiences all the time. These exist in the mind as abstract forms, and are not inextricably bound to a particular mode or even to the world of feelings at all – and it is these which permit us to experience a perceptually unified world. The vitality affects include the qualities of, e.g. surging, fading away, fleeting and drawn out (Stern 1985; Stern *et al.* 1985), and these are part of the way that we breathe, move, get hungry, wake up, get angry, feel sad, play tennis, or whatever. It is our internal, both bodily and affective, experiences of these vitality affects as infants, that give us a sense of the dynamic shifts and patterned changes of not only ourselves, but of how others are and how the world is. In terms of perceptual unity, we can understand the meaning of a child bursting with energy, a burst of temper, a burst watermelon, bursting into tears, a burst of speed, and so on. The 'bursting' is the qualitative form of the action or feeling, irrespective of whether it is a positive or negative emotion, or of whether there is any feeling component at all. In music we speak of a sforzando to illustrate that quality in a burst of sound.

As we shall see later, music can portray vitality affects by reproducing properties that belong not only to feelings, but to any movement, shape, contour and intensity. We recognise what Suzanne Langer calls the 'morphology' of music as having to do with our own emotional and perceptual life. In the next chapter, we shall see how music therapy improvisation generates and extends a person's vitality affects in the context of a relationship. Vitality affects enable us to make sense to one another.

Receiving the Other (or: Shall we Dance?)

What is becoming clear is that we not only communicate as cohesive beings, but, more critically, we perceive one another's acts as cohesive forms. Thus each partner in a communicating dyad perceives the other's acts as a temporally co-ordinated whole, rather than as disparate fragments of behaviour. In communicating with someone else, we do not simply see the shape of their smile or hear the inflection of their voice or the speed at which they move their hands: rather we perceive the totality of that person, and respond to this totality, which includes the various qualitative dimensions of themselves. This is consonant with earlier discussion on perceptual psychology, that showed our brains to be predisposed to patterning and to global perception, rather than to perceiving the world as a sum of parts.

Condon and Ogston (1966) describe the interlocking of motions and flows between the speaker and the listener as reinforcing and counterpointing one another. They write: 'Intensive analysis revealed harmonious or synchronous organisation of change between body motion and speech in *both* intra-individual and interactional behaviour. Thus, the body of the speaker dances in time with his speech. Further, the body of the listener dances in rhythm with that of the speaker' (p.338).

Intrasubjectivity and intersubjectivity

In order to achieve communication, the movements or acts of one human being must become a stimulus for the other: the motivation of the latter must be changed. The success of the communicating behaviour depends upon the individual's ability or capacity to read the communicative information which is carried by the movements or acts of the other person. Thus for effective communication between mother and infant, the infant must have the capacity to apprehend more than just the curve of the mother's mouth and the sounds that she makes: he must co-ordinate the two into a coherent form (a smile/her laughter), and be alert to what this tells him about how she is being with him. Stern (1985) writes: 'First, the parent must be able to 'read' the infant's mental state or inner experience from the infant's overt behaviour. Secondly, the infant must be able to 'read' this overt parental response as having to do with ('reflecting back,' etc.) his original experience' (p.249).

A new-born infant has the capacity to 'read' the mother's emotional signals in various modalities, i.e. her voice, gestures, movements and facial expressions, and to co-ordinate these disparate signals into a form which is meaningful for him, in that it conveys information about the mother's emotional state and its changes.

This may be illustrated by an example (cited in Pavlicevic 1990): a male infant moves his arm in such a way as to cause an object to flop about. This movement is perceived by the infant and by another person (e.g. his mother) to have a certain 'physiognomic' quality: it is irregular, quick and comes to an abrupt stop before suddenly jerking in another direction. These qualities reveal to the mother the infant's internal state of motivation. The mother apprehends, or 'reads', the form of the movement, i.e., its tempo, irregular rhythm and unexpected lengths of phrases, and may choose to express these qualities in her vocalisation which accompanies the infant's arm movement. Through apprehending the infant's forms, she has taken in a sense of his internal state and its change. The infant recognises the form of the mother's vocalisation as being related to his arm movement. He feels she has a feeling of how he feels. He then changes the quality of the movement, for example, he decreases the speed of his arm movement, expressing a variation in tempo, and then he awaits the corresponding change in his mother's voice. In this way, the infant learns about how his own alteration of form is perceived and reflected by another through vocal sounds. He explores the link of feeling between himself and his mother exchanged in different modalities. For this to happen, however, he is dependent upon his mother being sensitive to the emotion in the forms of his movement.

It is through sharing his feeling world with another – his mother – that the human infant defines and extends his sense of self-ness: he gains insight (or has his insight reinforced) into himself as an emotional and communicating human being, by experiencing his actions (and impulses to action) through his mother's response to them – whether she imitates, extends, complements or inverts them. The infant knows that she knows how he feels about their contact and their relationship.

The absence of this experience within the intimate association results in the infant failing to share aspects of himself with another, and may cause the infant to remain profoundly isolated or unrelated, emotionally and socially. Thus the quality of one's first relationship can be, or can be conceived as being, crucial in our learning about the world and ourselves within it (Bowlby 1969; Murray 1992; Stern 1985).

Knowing and interacting with another's internal state has been termed 'intersubjectivity' (Trevarthen 1980, 1986), and the mechanisms of the mother's adjustment of expression to match that of her infant 'affect attunement' (Stern 1985). When the partners' relationship is actively intersubjective, both infant and mother initiate, complement and respond to one another in a highly fluid and intimate dance, within which their internal states resonate with, and complement, one another.

This relating to one another continues throughout our lives, and continues to give us a sense of who we are and how the world is with us – so much so that it is well known that oppressive regimes use solitary confinement in order to 'break' people: by being isolated for a substantial period of time, we begin to lose sense of who we are.

Traditional sub-Saharan African cultures, which are highly group-oriented, speak of the concept of *Ubuntu*, which means something like, 'I exist because I see myself through you'. In other words, it is through my experience of myself through another that I have a sense of being alive. But in order to experience myself through another, I need to 'know' how they experience me. I need to know that their experience of me is authentic and genuine: I therefore need access to their internal states. Part of sharing our inner states with other people means experiencing our inner states as resonating with those of others. Most of us have the capacity to 'know' others and to know ourselves through their experience of us.

Disrupting the Dance

However, there are times when circumstances, genetics, chemical imbalances in our systems or environmental stresses, impinge on our capacity to 'share' and to 'resonate with' others in a fluid way. Here our capacity to resonate in a mutual, flowing intimacy with others is affected. If we are severely mentally ill, we may lose a sense of who we are, lose a sense of boundary between ourselves and 'the world' – we may experience a sense of personal disinte-gration, become invaded by 'foreign' voices, sounds and smells, and so on. All of these, of course, interfere with inter-personal fluency. Thus when Condon and Ogston (1966) compared (so-called) 'normal' adults commu-nicating, with a dyad where one partner suffered from a mental illness, the interactions between the latter pair were dyssynchronous. Condon and Ogston comment on the absence of mutual gaze-meeting patterns, in contrast to 'normal' interactions, the tense holding of the elements of posture in relation to one another (the normal sag of relaxed posture is missing), and the self-dyssynchrony which they did not find in their analysis of 'normal' behaviour. We have a sense, here, of the speaker and listener not reading and connecting with one another's vitality affects. Whereas in the optimal interaction the speaker and listener flowed together in a way that suggested a smooth receiving, encoding and transfer of one another's amodal qualities (i.e. the listener moving in time with the intonation of the speaker's voice), much in the same way that a baby moves in synchrony with the mother's voice, in the 'disturbed' dyad we see an absence of this, which is translated into unflowing, uncommunicative 'being with other'. Here we are reminded of Lynne Murray's work, where depressed mothers and their babies show a less synchronous engagement with one another (Murray and Trevarthen 1986; Murray and Stein 1991). We shall see later that these dyssynchronous mechanisms are portrayed in clinical improvisations in music therapy.

Many of us have, at one or other time, experienced feelings of depression: our movements slow down, the energy and volition of our acts diminishes, and we may become 'flat' in our affect. Any one of these influences how we respond to others. We find it difficult to 'flow' with them at their tempo, dynamic level, etc., and unable to negotiate a mutual fluency; we remain lagged and unresponsive. People who have suffered from strokes and brain injuries may lose their pre-accident fluidity and congruence of being, and need to make enormous adaptations to re-experience themselves in this new mode. All too often, a secondary feature of many disabilities, whether mental or physical, or of pathologies, neurological injuries and so on, is the profound experience of isolation. This isolation can be the result of something as simple as not being able to speak quickly enough, not having the emotional volition to laugh, not having enough movement control to gesture, and so on. The person is unable to engage with others in a confluent mode, and remains excluded from intimate human rapport. As a result of this, they may gain a distorted sense of who they are – or who they have become. For example, I was once asked to do a one-off music therapy group session with a group of stroke patients who attended a weekly social club. I recall clearly my initial and instant impression of 'slowness'. Everything took a long time. When we were finally ready to play, the playing tempo was slow: I had to slow down my natural, rather upbeat tempo in order for us to meet in the music. Even within the music, it took a long time for me to begin to flow in what had, at first, felt like an unnatural and uncomfortable pace. It took a long time for us to begin to 'dance' together.

Interactional Synchrony

It is apparent that while reading the coherent temporal structures of the other person, we ourselves are not merely passive recipients of information about them. We ourselves move our being, whether in speech, movement, posture or facial expressions, in sympathy with them. Condon and Ogston (1966) have shown that when two people speak to one another, not only does the speaker's body move in synchrony with their speech, but, concurrently, the listener's body moves in synchrony with the speaker's speech, so that what occurs is a subtly fluctuating dance between listener and speaker. This phenomenon has been called 'interactional synchrony' (Brown and Avstreih 1989).

As communicating persons, we attune to much more than the verbal content of what is being said – there is a stream of communicative acts that is immensely powerful and immediate in conveying how we experience one another and ourselves within the context of verbally based communication. These acts are as immediate and powerful as the semantics being exchanged through words.

Feldstein and Welkowitz (1978) have demonstrated that a high degree of empathy, or emotional rapport, between conversing adults can be observed the closer they adapt and adjust the prosodic elements of their speech to one another. In other words, they 'tune in' to one another by beginning to mirror the dynamic level (or loudness) of their speech, the length of their phrases, the timbre of their speaking voice, and so on. Feldstein and Welkowitz emphasise the psychological importance of timing in interactive acts: the interacting partners' pacing, duration and timing of their spoken utterances reveal both characteristic patterns of the individual and the quality of their interaction. Adults characteristically show an inclination towards what they call 'congruence': speakers develop interpersonal influence with regard to intensity and durational values of utterances in their conversations.

Bernieri and Rosenthal (1991) draw our attention to the fact that interpersonal co-ordination is present in nearly all aspects of our social lives. We are all intimately – and biologically – linked to our environment. This environment, they suggest, is periodic and our bodies are 'captured' by its cycles. In this sense the environment is a 'time-giver', to which our physio-logical processes synchronise. The authors use the word 'entrainment' to describe this capturing of our bodies rhythms by external cycles. However, we also synchronise to social cues: thus we are entrained not just to climate and temperature, but also to other persons, synchronising our behaviour cycles to them, with periods of engagement and disassociation. The authors draw from a substantial body of literature suggesting that, within an interacting dyad, the time-giver may be the dominant partner of the relationship. In other words, interpersonal matching is not only a feature of early years. Bernieri and Rosenthal describe interpersonal co-ordination as, '...the degree to which behaviours in an interaction are non-random, patterned or synchronised, in both timing and form' (p.403).

Interactional synchrony is composed of rhythm, simultaneous movement and the smooth meshing of interaction, and a feature of this interpersonal co-ordination is that of matching. Where the physiological behaviour of two persons is congruent, they are believed – and judged – to have a higher rapport with one another than two persons whose postures are less similar. Their inter-personal co-ordination is seen as reflecting their internal affective states and their attitudes to one another.

Thus we see that communicative forms exist within all of us, and they are flexible in terms of energy and contour: we may speak quickly, loudly, in a staccato manner and, correspondingly, our movements and gestures will reflect these qualitative aspects of our speech. Their existence enables us to read the temporal flexibility or fluidity of these patterns in others, enables us to respond flexibly and to complement one another's gestures, facial expressions and vocalisations. They enable us to be in tune with other human beings. In music therapy improvisation, we tune in to the quality of this energy and create a relationship through sound forms that highlights these very qualities.

Matching and Mis-Matching

Daniel Stern makes the point that when the correspondence between mother and infant is well matched, the infant frequently reacts by not reacting, e.g. the infant may continue as though nothing has happened, expressing self-satisfied pleasure in communication. However, when there is a mis-matching, when, for example, the mother over-attunes or under-attunes to the infant's action, the infant's reaction communicates to his mother an alertness to this, e.g. he may stop the activity and look at her with puzzlement. Stern (1985) relates a delightful example of observing an infant who is crawling along the ground, being jigged by his mum in tempo to his crawling. To everyone's surprise he continues to crawl as though nothing were happening, apparently ignoring his mum. The psychologists then suggest to her that she jigs him 'out of time' with his crawling – she does this and the infant instantly looks up at her with a puzzled expression. But to what is she over- or under-attuning? To the qualities of shape, intensity, time and motion – the amodal properties that we all recognise and tune into. The baby knows that there is a disjunction in the interactional synchrony between itself and its mother.

Various psychologists, such as Tronick *et al.* (1979) and Papousek and Papousek (1981), have commented on the quality of a mother's mis-match-ing. They propose that in a sensitive mother, the quality or degree of mis-matching will not be beyond her baby's capabilities, and will offer him a more complex and expanded environment in which to grow. A consistently perfectly matched environment, although enhancing communication at that moment, would not provide for growth. The paediatrician and psychoanalyst Winnicott makes a similar point when he talks about the inherent frustration of growing older: the mother does not always act or react as though she were an extension of the infant (Winnicott 1971). Although this irritates and frustrates the child, it also provides him with an environment with just the right degree of unpredictability or uncertainty, into which he needs to expand in order to continue developing.

Lynne Murray's studies with infants of 6–12 weeks, have shown that when mothers grossly mis-match their expression to the expression of their infants, the infants show signs of distress. They try to attract the mothers' attention and eventually become withdrawn. Murray also showed that the quality of babies' attention towards their mothers alters depending on the nature of her mis-matching. Thus when the mothers' attention was distracted by a person entering the room, the babies remained relaxed and undistressed, their attention to their mothers decreased and they looked at the new person. However, when the interruption was caused by the mothers assuming a 'blank face condition', where under the researcher's instruction they ceased to respond altogether, the babies' efforts to communicate with their mothers increased for a time, they showed signs of distress and finally became

withdrawn and uncommunicative (Murray 1988, 1992; Murray and Trevarthen 1985).

Revisiting Clinical Improvisation

What does all of this have to do with music therapy improvisation, we might
ask. First, we can see that the elements of music, i.e., pulse, rhythm, pitch,
timbre and volume, can be abstracted from our expressive acts and transferred
across modalities, organised and combined in a way that re-creates, through
sound, the intensity and shape and motion of both self- and interactional-
synchrony. Spontaneous music improvisation can portray smoothness, fluidity or interruptions and distortions of our being as they are happening within
an interaction. The musical portrayal of our capacity for self-organisation is
not an artificial or inauthentic leap into 'art form'. Rather it would seem that
music is, in any case, a fundamental part of our social experiences from an
early age. In this sense, formal musical instruction may be seen as a stylised,
inauthentic distortion of a natural 'music'.

Thus when I was improvising with Noel (Chapter 2), my experience of
playing with him was that the music was portraying *him in relation to me*. I
did not experience the music as a solitary *musical* event, i.e. as only 'his' music,
but as portraying both his capacity for self-co-ordination and for self- and
interactional-synchrony. It was through this shared portrayal and experience
that I was able to get a sense of who and how Noel is in the world. Moreover,
this self- and interactional-co-ordination was experienced, not simply as a
co-ordination of movements (in the way that the two argumentative cats were
described), but as conveying something about his inner life, about the
flexibility and adaptability of his vitality affects – the nature of energy,
fluidity and motion in his feeling life. Thus his 'tight busy-ness' was not just
musical, it was about him: how he lives, how he engages, how he expresses
and experiences himself *in relation to*. 'This is me', he said after playing.

If, as we have seen, musical elements underpin our emotional, expressive
life as well as the way that we receive and give communication to others,
both as infants and adults, then we see that disorders in any of these realms
will have musical correspondences. Disturbances in communication may be
seen – and experienced directly – through disturbances in the timing,
sequencing, amplitude, energy and fluidity of acts and gestures, as well as in
disruptions of inter-co-ordinating acts with another person. We saw earlier
that when we are depressed, we find it difficult to 'flow' with others and
remain slow, flat and monotonic. Those who engage with us will experience
a measure of discomfort at our lack of responsiveness or flexibility. From
both their own discomfort and from their direct experience of the subtle (or

not so subtle) absence or distortion of interactional synchrony, they will infer that we are 'not with it'.

Musicians know that timing, periodicity, sequencing, texture and phrasing are parts of the musical vocabulary, and an interruption or distortion of any of these in musical performance often results in the musician being considered 'unmusical'. Music therapists, however, have direct experience, through jointly created clinical improvisation, of distorted inter-timing, interrupted fluidity and collapsed reciprocity in the improvisation, and here these signal not a lack of musicality, but, because of the interpersonal context, an interpersonal dyssynchrony.

In music therapy improvisation when the music therapist and client cannot generate a smooth musical interplay with one another, this usually suggests various interactional dynamics: the therapist may be having an 'off' day and is unable to meet or match the client; she may not be concentrating; the client may be unwilling – at an unconscious level – to engage with the therapist; the client may have a reduced emotional capacity to engage with another, or the client may have a neurological or physical basis for the absence of 'smoothness', although this is a different matter altogether. Any one of these – and other – dynamics are portrayed by the musical interplay. Music therapy gives relational meaning to these disturbances and distortions.

Thus clinical improvisation attempts to 'read' the client's capacity to organise themselves in order to enter into communication with another person: for example, is the client 'organised' until the therapist joins in, and at that moment becomes chaotic? Or is the client rigidly organised, showing no sign of acknowledging the therapist in the music, but remaining, rather, a closed, perseverating system? Parallel to this, the improvisation checks whether the client is able to 'read' the communicative and expressive features of the music, or does the client merely see the musical event as itself? For example, in working with patients who suffered from chronic schizophrenia, I noticed that their comments after the improvisations were often concrete: they might comment on whether they liked or did not like the music, on whether it was 'nice' or not, but even when asked directly, they seemed almost never to read the clinical improvisation as anything other than just music, remaining apparently unaware of its fuller significance. In contrast depressed patients, or emotionally distressed patients, grasped that this was *not* about 'playing music', almost immediately. This was, at times, a source of stress and anxiety about playing music, and the person might verbalise something like, 'what can you tell about me from the way I play?'

When music therapy improvisation is able to generate an inter-personal context between therapist and client, then the improvisation elicits and portrays the client's experience of himself-in-the-world, through sound. This is in contrast to the amodal and the cross-modal experience of the world, where we might gesture, move or speak in order to convey something about ourselves. In music therapy we invite clients to engage predominantly through music – through sound. In fact we might say that we elicit and respond to the clients 'mono-modally', instead of through all of the modalities of everyday expression. To return to Robarts' description, Colin screams, drums his feet on the floor, and hurtles towards a temper tantrum – he is expressing himself multi-modally. The therapist reads his various acts (vocal, facial, motor) as being 'musical', and acknowledges this 'musicality' not through her own multi-modal acts, but through sound form. For example, the tension of his acts: the one tension that is conveyed through his various modalities, is matched by the therapist through the modality of sound. This sound form, which is the channel of communication, refers to the amodal quality of the child's multi-modal acts, and this quality is, I suggest, the 'essential' child: this quality is what Nordoff and Robbins mean by the 'music' child. This does not ignore the fact that the act of creating sound form is in itself multi-modal. The therapist moves, gathers the whole of herself in order to create this sound form: but the pivot, the focus, is the sounds. Robarts describes the 'glissandi', the 'tonality' of his screams and the foot-drumming as 'conversational'. Through the sound forms, the therapist and child 'converse'.

In listening to Nordoff and Robbins' (1977) audio recording of their work with Edward, the tape amply conveys the developing relationship between the therapists and the child – despite the absence of a picture of the child. In this sense, video recordings of sessions may distract from the essential sound form – although showing that vitality affects are, after all, cross-modal.

Thus the client's playing may show – and, indeed, ought to show – a corresponding intensity in posture and facial expression. But what if the opposite happens? In working with a complicated middle-aged woman who suffered from a mental illness, her body posture was almost foetal, coy, turned inwards. The music revealed an intensity and extroverted passion that made for one of those magical music therapy experiences: this quiet, rather helpless woman was a smouldering volcano! It was as though the full complement of her expressiveness was channelled through the music. The joint music improvisation captured and displayed the vitality affects that she seemed to hide. What she typically conveyed and expressed through speech, gestures and movement was a rather sorrowful, pathetic and helplessly dependent person.

We can say that in music therapy, one of the therapist's tasks is to 'read' the vitality affects of the person as these are elicited in the joint clinical improvisation. The therapist, however, does more than 'read' them: she is also directly involved: she has direct experience of the client's feeling states, through playing with the client, in a manner that seeks to create an intersubjective experience for therapist and client. The client has a sense that the therapist 'knows' how the client feels. The therapist, too, through this direct experience, gets a clear sense of the patient's 'core self', i.e., how the client experiences himself, and acts, in the world. The therapeutic work, then, is meeting and matching the client's music in order to give the client an experience of 'being known', through his sounds being responded to as being expressively and communicatively meaningful, rather than as the client playing music – and, further, developing this engagement through sustained, joint improvisations.

The next chapter turns the mirror the other way, by exploring the communicative and expressive mechanisms of clinical improvisation through the theoretical framework of non-verbal communication.

CHAPTER 9

Music in Dynamic Form
and Dynamic Form in Music

We have seen, by now, that musicality is innate. This musicality is part of our earliest engagements, part of our ongoing expressive and communicative life. Musicality, in this sense, is not about being 'musically talented'.

This innate musicality, often subsumed by the emergence, and eventual primacy, of words is tapped in music therapy, precisely because its essential nature is emotional. Thus when Nordoff and Robbins (1977) speak of 'the music child', the music to which they refer is a part of our relating, emotional life. Music therapy improvisation addresses 'the music child' – by inviting the person to express him or herself through sounds and by reading the child/adult's capacity for flexibility in organising rhythm, melody, tempo – as portraying the person expressive and communicative, reciprocal capacities. In clinical work, however, it is usually the distortion of this innate musicality that is addressed, that points the way towards how the person can be brought towards a state of equilibrium and balanced flexibility, signalling a fully mutual expressive being. The person's autism/depression/handicap/difficulty has been amply documented and classified by experts. For the music therapist, it is the *quality* of the person's innate, and relating, musicality that sounds volumes.

Increasingly of late, music therapy literature is acknowledging this body of knowledge on non-verbal communication as one of the theoretical paradigms underpinning music therapy (Bunt 1994; Hughes 1995; Oldfield 1995; Pavlicevic 1990, 1991, 1994, 1995a, 1996b; Robarts 1994, 1996). However, we need to be clear about which aspects of this literature are appropriate, and we need to be cautious not to make too literal a comparison. A non-verbal dialogue between a (verbally competent) mother and a newborn infant (who is verbally naive) cannot comfortably be compared with that between a music therapist (who is a highly skilled musician) and a client, who may – or may not – be a skilled musician. In music therapy, both partners may be verbally competent, so that the therapist and client need not, in fact, relate through non-words. However, in music therapy, the primary mode for relating is that of sound, and this must have some impact on the nature of the interaction. Here the partners know that they can 'hop out' of the music and into words if they wish. In an interaction between mother and infant, there is no choice about being non-verbal: that is the only available resource to the dyad.

Some of the music therapy literature that draws from mother–infant interaction is not altogether convincing, and this reinforces the arguments of those music therapists who discourage music therapists from applying theories from a different, if allied, discipline, on the grounds that one paradigm cannot comfortably be transposed on to another (Aigen 1991; Ansdell 1995; Lee, op.cit.). Certainly some careful teasing out needs to be done, in order to clarify what concepts are useful and what can be left behind.

For example, I found Heal's comparison of a music therapy session involving an adult mentally handicapped person with a mother interacting with a four-week-old baby, albeit from a psychoanalytic position, somewhat incomplete (Hughes 1995). We know from psychoanalytic theory, that the quality of our life experiences as adults is grounded in our primary emotional experiences, so that, for example, the feelings of loss that Heal's client experiences no doubt have their root in earlier experiences of loss. However, I remain dissatisfied with the inferred parallels between the baby sucking her thumb (as a substitute for the breast) and the client's spinning of the cymbal in the music therapy session (as a way of coping with emotions around loss). In reading the text, it felt rather as though the writer experi-enced similar feelings in the two situations, and was able, through that, to make connections between them – *for herself.* This is entirely valid as a clinical observation, in the sense that all therapists rely on personal insights and feelings for their clinical information. However, the fact that the same or similar feelings were elicited in both situations does not necessarily mean that the two situations are comparable to quite the extent suggested in the text. My concern is that by not teasing out carefully what does and does not belong to the music therapy situation, we may complicate the meaning of events in sessions.

More practically helpful to music therapists, I think, is the thinking of Leslie Bunt (1994) and Amelia Oldfield (1995), both of whom offer descriptions of communicative mechanisms between mother and infants, and draw direct observational (rather than inferential) comparisons between these and the music therapy interaction. In Oldfield's discussion, the fine line in a music therapy session between the therapist being directive, and thereby anticipating certain responses from the child, and the therapist allowing the child the freedom to respond in any which way, is directly compared with a mother and baby cooing and gurgling to one another, with the mother adapting her vocal sounds in order to allow the baby space to respond. This does not necessarily mean that the music therapy situation re-creates the early mother–infant situation for the client.

Leslie Bunt (1994) goes further, exploring in detail communicative features such as turn-taking, waiting, imitating and responding, in child–adult interactions and in music therapy sessions. He draws comparisons between the imitative behaviour of a young infant, who is learning to share a language and object world, with adults, and the imitation in music therapy with children. According to Bunt, imitation in music therapy is a more passive response from the child, which precedes a more active, initiating mode. Turn-taking patterns that are present in pre-verbal, synchronous interactions between adults and infants make use of interactive features, such as silences and switch-over points, that are similar to those found when a therapist is being sensitive to the child's musical patterns, inviting the child to develop skills of communicating intentions to the adult, and responding to the adult's intent.

Robarts (1996) explains clearly in her interpretation of the work with Colin, that the musical acts create the potential relationship. She uses tone, rhythm, and tempo to match or enhance Colin's vocal sounds, movements or gestures darwing clear and direct associations between the boy's musical acts and her own, and what these mean in terms of the therapeutic relationship.

All of these descriptions help to clarify where and why therapy happens in music, but the essential link between our musical and our emotional life in the context of music therapy improvisation still needs to be explicated. I now want to explore the concept of 'Dynamic Form' in music therapy, which has been written about elsewhere (Pavlicevic 1990, 1991, 1994, 1995a, 1996b), since this concept underpins explanations as to why musical behaviour may be read as emotional or relational behaviour in the first instance. This discussion purposely omits psychodynamic concepts in order not to complicate the concepts set out below.

Dynamic Form of Music and Emotion

The concept of Dynamic Form takes root from the intrinsically organised dynamic forms of emotions which are present from birth and generated in interpersonal relating, whether between a mother and infant or between relating adults. These dynamic forms of feeling exist as abstract functional entities in the mind and are signalled through the qualities of our expressive acts. In music therapy, these may be signalled through the expressive quality of musical improvisation, e.g., those of tempo (accellerando, rubato, ritardando), dynamics (sforzando, crescendo) or modulations of timbre and pitch – where an intersubjective, musical context is generated. Dynamic Form, in this sense, does not exist separately from the musical relationship between therapist and client, neither does it exist as separate from the music: Dynamic Form is signalled exclusively through the music that is spontaneously improvised by the therapist and client. The quality of the Dynamic Form indicates the quality of the relationship between the therapist and client, and this in turn indicates the client's (and the therapist's, of course) capacity for forming an intimate, intersubjective relationship with another.

We saw earlier that Daniel Stern's (1985) concept of vitality affects captures the amodality or cross-modality of feeling form. This concept offers one explanation as to why and how we use music improvisation in music therapy. A critical point is that vitality affects are elicited within an *interactive* context. They are not static states that exist in an unengaged, solitary mind. Another critical point is that here, although thinking of music as an 'emotional' relationship, we are not thinking of emotion as being the *external* display of internal, categorical emotional states such as joy, anger, sadness, and so on, which is the traditional view of emotion, both in psychology and in music aesthetics. Rather vitality affects pertain to the underlying, non-referential dynamic processes that can be seen as underpinning categorical emotional states. Thus a vitality affect of, say, smoothness and tightness can be a quality that is part of being angry, of being sad, of being frustrated or of being pleased – and the musical relationship seeks to elicit and extend this quality.

The significance of clinical improvisation is that it is an *inter-personal* event, rather than only being a *musically* interactive event. The improvisation creates a quality of engagement that reveals personal (rather than just musical) qualities about the two (or more) individuals that partake in – and create – the improvisation. Through the quality of the joint improvisation, the therapist and client learn about one another. This does not, however, mean that a joint improvisation whose focus is musical, rather than interactive, will elicit this intimacy and interpersonal knowing. The critical distinction between a purely musical improvisation and one that happens to use music in order to create an 'interpersonal engagement' can be understood by the concept of Dynamic Form.

Dynamic Form corresponds to Daniel Stern's vitality affects, but is explicitly musical in character. Vitality affects are properties of feelings as well as of music, and involve amodal properties of shape, contour, intensity level, motion, number and rhythm, that may be expressed through any of the senses. A shape may be large, small, narrow, broad; a contour can be smooth, fluid, jerky, broken; intensity can be a sudden increase, a gradual build-up, it can remain static for a while and suddenly change; motion can be quick or slow, it can fluctuate, it can turn around, go backwards, sideways or whatever; number, surely, needs no explanation; and rhythm may be smooth and lulling, impulsive or compulsive, or it can be fragmented and unsettled. These amodal properties are part of our cognitive, neurological and perceptual capacities, and they are signalled through the qualities of our expressive acts. Thus we can have a mental idea of interacting with someone who is fast, mercurial, changeable, because we have experienced this quality in playing with a lively kitten or in watching a blob of mercury move around a container. Or we can describe music as rough and prickly, because we have an experience, or a mental image, of a hedgehog, a prickly pear or of someone with a 'prickly' personality. These are amodal properties, and they are cross-modal in the sense that any of these qualities can belong to any of our modalities: we can speak quickly in a staccato way, we can move in the same way, we can gesticulate and grimace in a quick staccato way, and we recognise quick, staccato music.

The duality of musical and emotional processes in clinical improvisation is illustrated in Figure 9.1. Here the y-axis represents the range of communication that is possible between two persons, from non-interaction, where each partner is isolated from the other, through to a high degree of mutuality, with close interaction and a mutually satisfying, reciprocal relationship. The x-axis represents contrasting limitations and restrictions of the emotional/musical events. Here fragmented playing is contrasted with a highly organised, rigid mode of expression. In considering these limitations/potentials, we are thinking not just of how someone spontaneously 'plays' music, but of how they are 'in the world'. The one is read as the other. For example, fragmented musical utterances of one partner make it more difficult for the second partner to join in with them: the second partner struggles to make sense of these utterances, not just at a perceptual/cognitive level, as we saw in Chapters 5 and 6, but also in a relational sense. To put it verbally: how can I talk with you when your words are all jumbled up and I cannot make sense of what you say? Similarly, a rigid and perseverative musical form with little fluctuation severely limits how the two partners play together: their Dynamic Form is limited, narrow – and their relating remains restricted. This perseverativeness and rigidity tell the therapist something about how the client expresses him or herself.

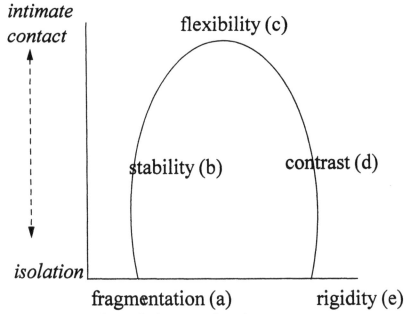

Figure 9.1 Dynamic form in the therapeutic relationship

The inverted U shows that where the client reveals 'fragmentation and disorder' (a), which means that his or her world is potentially isolated, the therapist needs to 'lead' or 'invite' the client towards stability (b), in order to potentiate the beginnings of a relationship between them. Her conscious – and rather calculated – musical move is termed a 'clinical intervention': in this example she may offer the client a stable pulse, in order to provide him or her with the stability so lacking in his or her playing. Often, though, the client's lack of emotional integration results in a flip-over into perseverative rigidity (e): here, the Dynamic Form is brittle and unsteady. It cannot yet move towards flexibility, via stability. All too often, rigidity and chaotic playing are a flip-side of the same coin: that of isolation.

If, in contrast, the improvisation's Dynamic Form is rigidly organised and perseverative (e), the therapist may, as a clinical intervention, offer music with 'contrast' (d), thereby offering an extension of the Dynamic Form towards which the client can grow. Here, again, my experience of working with chronically ill schizophrenic patients was that the move towards flexibility of Dynamic Form – and towards a more intimate relationship – was a tortuous one, with constant spills into fragmentation and disorder, at which point the therapist would offer stability and risk the client flipping into perseveration, and so on. The attempt to generate flexibility often passed through both, polarised, modes of playing.

How, though, does the therapist musically elicit the Dynamic Form in the first instance? How does she extend it? What happens 'inside' an improvisation?

Let us imagine that a client begins to play spontaneously on a bass drum. The therapist listens and, within the first moments, establishes the quality of shape, intensity and motion of the client's playing. This is revealed in the intensity of energy of the beat, whether this is sustained or erratic; in the quality of the beating's motion, whether it is regular, whether the regularity is stuck, compulsive, whether there is a flexibility about it, and so on. The therapist will be alert to the quality of the pulse, or basic beat, of the client's playing. We can conceptualise this as the therapist listening for a potential invariant which, as we saw earlier, is one of the mechanisms that helps us to make sense of our environment. In this instance we can think of pulse, or the basic beat, as the 'primary' relational invariant. Nordoff and Robbins (1977, p.134) write: 'The basic beat is the foundation of musical-rhythmic order, the underlying time base of coherent musical activity and experience'. The basic beat may be thought of as the basis upon which the relationship can be built.

In listening to the client's opening musical utterances, the therapist gauges whether or not she can begin improvising in such a manner as to create a musical relationship with the client. This relationship, however, is not one-sided: while beginning, cautiously, to play, she will at the same time be alert to the client's response to her playing and may modify what she does, taking the client's response into account. At the same time the client may be listening to the therapist's playing, and modify his or her playing according to what the client hears. In this way a swift and subtle, constantly shifting relationship begins to develop, with both partners taking cues from one another and affecting one another's music. But what are the mechanisms used? How do they do it?

Let us go back to the opening moments. When the therapist begins to play, she may use one of three rhythmic mechanisms for meeting the client, which I would like to crystallise. Music combines rhythm, melody, pitch, timbre and so on, but in clarifying these mechanisms I discuss them from a rhythmic perspective: melody, in any case, includes rhythm and rhythm includes timbre as well as dynamic level, so that while focusing on the players' rhythmic components, I should like this to contain other ingredients. Also, since at times it is the client that may mirror the therapist, I have labelled the players 'neutrally', 'A' and 'B'.

Mirroring, Matching, Reflecting

Let us assume, for the moment, that there is a regular pulse in A's playing, even if its quality may be highly implicit. B hears this pulse and begins to play in a manner that meets A. How does B meet A?

Mirroring signifies that one partner (A) imitates the other (B) strictly and concurrently, as though the two were facing each other in a musical mirror. The first partner literally does what the second partner does, at the same time. This is not 'imitation', which implies a time-lag, but a concurrent, synchronous event, where the two players travel together, illustrated in Figure 9.2. Mirroring implies that A's playing is predictable, and that B can join in, coincidentally. If A is playing a melodic instrument, which means that her patterns have a melodic component as well as a rhythmic one, then B can mirror this pattern rhythmically, either on an untuned percussion instrument or else by playing a melodic instrument in such a way as to resonate harmonically with what A is doing. In mirroring, the partners' accents coincide, they share a sense of the metre of the music.

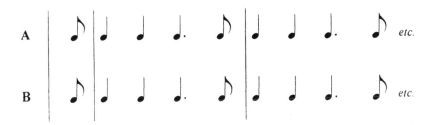

Figure 9.2 Mirroring

Mirroring may signify various relational aspects, depending on when and how it occurs. For example, where therapist and client have been circling one another, not quite managing to connect through the music, and then arrive at a moment of mirroring, this is a moment of connectedness where the partners are doing the same thing at the same time. This moment may be defined by previous relational instabilities or differences between them. Although the musical content of this moment of mirroring may be pedestrian and rather banal, the *relational* significance of this moment is important: it opens the doors for both partners, allowing each one to be with the other. Another example of the significance of mirroring may come at the end of a long and complex improvisation, where suddenly, as though by magic, both players end quickly, without 'approaching' the ending. My experience of this kind of event is that it is tremendously exciting, by its unexpectedness, and that it may be an indication of a closer, tighter relationship where the players seem almost to divine one another's intentions, however unexpected these might be.

The two partners, however, do not always play the same thing at the same time. Musical contact is not that literal, and if it were, we would question its relational quality. The partners also meet one another through the mechanism of *matching*. Here some, but not all, of the rhythmic components are mirrored (Figure 9.3). Matching can be thought of as partial mirroring where, for example, A plays a definite and predictable musical pattern, and B mirrors some, but not all, of the rhythmic components.

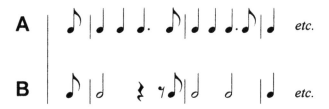

Figure 9.3 Matching

In clinical improvisation, the therapist may use this mechanism as a clinical tool, when the client's patterns are rigidly repetitive, and the therapist begins to provide only partial support and an alternative pattern at the same time. If the client detects the alternative musical form, he or she may begin to mirror the therapist, who may then provide the client with yet another alternative, by moving from mirroring to matching, and so on. In terms of Dynamic Form, the therapist may gradually begin to introduce an extension of Dynamic Form, inviting the client to extend themselves towards a broader, expressive sound form.

In thinking about the mechanism of *reflecting* we see that this can have various relational implications. Reflecting occurs when, for example, the players share a pulse but not a metric sense of the music. Here aspects of musical patterns pass from one player to the other, but not at the same time (Figure 9.4). If we think of a spectrum of relationship between the players, from low to high contact, then we see that reflecting may occur at a low level of contact where, for example, A's playing is unpredictable, so that B, in attempting to meet A, always feels that she is lagging behind, reproducing aspects of A's playing later in the improvisation.

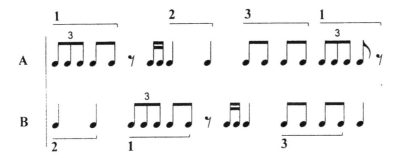

Figure 9.4 Reflecting

There is a clear example of this in work that I did with an adult woman: in our first session I was unsettled, not quite 'attuned' to her, and my playing portrayed this. In listening to the tape recording I hear that my improvisation changes tack every few moments, and the poor woman is trying to catch up, while at the same time trying to do her own improvisation. The example is a hit-and-miss affair, with each of us at times reflecting aspects of one another's playing. This improvisation did not manage to elicit an authentic Dynamic Form, since the therapist was 'not there' – the resulting brittleness in Dynamic Form needed to be revised in later sessions, when the therapist was a little more attuned to the client (and to herself).

However, reflecting may also denote a high level of musical contact, where the players know one another and trust one another to such an extent that they do not have to show it. Here the pulse of the music may be highly implicit, and the improvisation is 'loose' in the sense that, as a whole, it makes total musical sense, even though each of the players seems constantly to give and take various aspects of the music. This is a highly flexible, fluid and shareable Dynamic Form, where the partners are so 'in tune' that they can be idiosyncratic, musically, not follow the rules and yet 'know' one another. In an improvisation with a musician colleague, which formed part of a pilot project, our joint playing was quite chaotic and fragmented, with bits of rhythms here and there – and yet we both knew where we were: our connection was 'tight' – and on detailed listening to the recording, almost the entire improvisation uses the mechanism of reflecting – although here the reflecting is subtle and at a micro-level.

In terms of a clinical intervention, the therapist may use the tool of reflecting with a client who is musically over-dependent, always imitating the therapist, always following. The therapist may need to become less predictable in order to suggest, through the music, an alternate way of being.

These images of musical relationships are created here with the focus on rhythm. However, a child's crying sounds, and indeed his stamping of feet, also portray qualities of shape, intensity and motion that the therapist may begin to reproduce through improvisation, creating a Dynamic Form that is reflecting the shape, intensity and motion of the child's crying; or she may tap a hand-drum, matching the shape, tempo and intensity of the child's expressive gestures and acts. Here Dynamic Form is generated despite the therapist playing 'alone' – she is, of course, not playing alone. Her playing takes into account not only the other person, but also her feelings about the other person. She is not merely creating a 'musical impression' of the child's mood, but is directly engaging with the child.

In a paper on group improvisation (Pavlicevic 1995b) I alluded to the fact that the music in music therapy is not always 'sounded': it may exist in its unsounded form (as in the rather esoteric concept of the 'unstruck chord'). Despite earlier assertions that Dynamic Form is inseparable from the jointly created musical-emotional relationship between therapist and client (Pavlicevic 1996b), I would like to propose, tentatively, that Dynamic Form may be unrealised in the early stages of music therapy sessions. By this I mean that through the client's (non-musical) acts, the therapist may get a sense of the client's expressive qualities and, therefore, a *potential* sense of the Dynamic Form as yet unrealised through music. If we return to Robarts' description of Colin hurtling towards a tantrum in the first session, we see the therapist matching and reflecting aspects of his acts through her musical acts. Here she is setting the scene for Dynamic Form, drawing from the quality of who and how the child is, and letting the child have a sense of her 'knowing' him through her sounds.

In clinical improvisation, then, musical sounds have more than a musical function: they have a psychological, communicative function, in the sense that we do not simply improvise music with someone in order to 'play music', in the same way that mothers and infants do not vocalise just in order to make musical sounds. This may be illustrated by a project in which Sandra Brown and I attempted to clarify how, if both the music therapist and the client are highly skilled musicians, we know that they are not just 'making music' together (Brown and Pavlicevic 1996). In using ourselves as guinea pigs, and while aware of (and apprehensive about) the personal risks involved in taking turns at using ourselves as 'subjects', we undertook three sessions with one another. In the first two sessions, we took turns at being therapist and client (i.e., in the first session, I was therapist and Sandra was client, and in the second session we reversed roles). In the third session we played together as musicians. We asked 'blind listeners' to listen to recordings of three improvisations, to identify which of the improvisations were 'clinical' and which were 'musical', and to give us their reasons for making these choices.

In listening to the audio recordings of the sessions, our blind raters – who were music therapists – were able to distinguish between sessions in which the improvisation was therapeutic, and the session in which the two players were 'making music'. How could they tell the difference? The raters reported being able to hear how and where, in the 'music therapy' sessions, the improvisation 'changed track' in order for the therapist to support and be with the client's idiosyncratic utterances. In the 'music' session, they heard the improvisation being dictated by the music – the improvisation followed a musical path, with switches and changes which were 'musical', rather than 'personal'. One of the blind raters, however, questioned the authenticity of the players 'swapping roles'. This made us reflect on the validity of what we were doing, and we agreed, after some soul-searching, that we do in fact 'swap roles' in our daily lives, at times being therapists, at times being 'clients' in our own analytic/therapeutic processes, and at times being 'musicians' who play for fun. This small study highlights another aspect of Dynamic Form: that we – all of us – are able to switch from playing 'just' music to Dynamic Form playing. In the former, aspects of ourselves are, inevitably, portrayed – and this is, after all, what distinguishes one performer from another. The primacy, here, is the musical meaning: we gather ourselves in order to give the optimal musical rendering. In the latter we are being ourselves in the world, engaging with it. The primacy here is the personal: we portray who and how we are in the world – through sound. This is, after all, what we expect and encourage music therapy clients to do in music therapy. Here we might think of ourselves as 'gathering the music', in order for it to 'play us'. Of course this latter statement treats music as something out there, that can be picked up and used by the players when needed – and this is precisely what Dynamic Form is not. Dynamic Form is ourselves, portrayed in relation to another, through sound.

It is this Dynamic Form that the music therapist 'reads', and both client and therapist experience directly, in clinical improvisation. We saw in Figure 9.1 that the music therapy improvisation is 'read' by the therapist for its *personally* relational, rather than its *musically* relational, qualities. The improvisation reveals how motivated the person is to engage with another, and this has nothing to do with how musical the person is. In fact, in work with adults there may be, at times, anxieties on the part of the client about playing music, often framed by the client as 'being unmusical' and about not being able to play. At times these anxieties have to do with the client sensing that the improvisation is, in fact, not about music but about themselves, and their lack of access to musical vocabulary can create a myth that they will reveal something about themselves which only the therapist will understand and detect. This, unsurprisingly, may make the client feel powerless and out of control.

There is an inherent paradox in the concept of Dynamic Form, since music and emotion (in the sense described above) are described as forming an interface, on one hand and, at the same time, as having a dual nature. This is because in music therapy, music and emotion share fundamental features: the one may be taken to represent the other – i.e. we hear the music, not as music but as dynamic feeling states. Thus the *musical* interaction displays reveal the *communicative* quality of the interaction and, conversely, non-musical acts such as gestures, movements, vocalisations and movements reveal musical, interactive features. It is in this sense that we can see music and emotion as having a common root, or as being one phenomenon with a dual nature. However, we need to be cautious: music and emotion are also separate areas of human experience, each with a rich and vast cultural, philosophical,

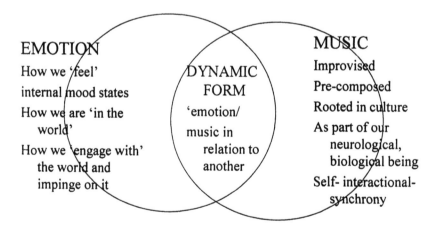

Figure 9.5 The dual nature of dynamic form shows the interface of music and emotion

literary and academic tradition. Their separateness is thus acknowledged by the concept of an interface (Figure 9.5), rather than suggesting that they merge totally and become one phenomenon: the interface symbolises that they share essential qualities and, at the same time, exist as separate phenomena. Thus the features of Dynamic Form are not purely musical, but then neither are they purely emotional.

In music therapy improvisation, it is the Dynamic Forms of the musical acts, as the partners relate to one another, rather than merely the separate, musical actions, that enable the therapist and client to know one another intimately. The inter-regulation of themselves in the music is more than the client merely 'playing music with' the therapist. For example, when the client imitates the therapist's music, the therapist assigns 'relational' meaning to this imitation: what is the client portraying by being constantly in imitative mode? An uncertainty about taking the initiative? A preference for letting someone else show the way? A state of dependency, or over-dependency, etc. etc. Meaning is multi-faceted and dynamic. The therapist and client are also not choosing to create music that is as musically interesting as possible: this would imply that the purpose of these inter-regulations was to learn the musical actions themselves, with the focus of the engagements remaining musical or on the surface. Again, if we 'read' the 'interesting' music interactively, then we can see that it may mean an avoidance of the 'personal' by remaining in the 'musical' sphere of interactivity. A parallel here is that mothers do not vocalise with infants in order to teach them to sing. Rather the inter-regulation of actions enables both partners to know that their subjective, internal state is intersubjectively shareable with, and knowable by, one another – their intentions, or impulses to act and feel, are reciprocated.

If we return once more to concepts from the literature on the intimate, intersubjective interaction between a mother and her infant, we can describe this fluid engagement as a 'dance'. This dance has all the complexities and subtleties of a musical improvisation duet which include expressive features of tempo, such as accelerando, rubato, ritardando, allargando and ritenuto; of dynamics, such as sforzando and crescendo; and emotionally coherent modulations of timbre and of pitch. If we look at music therapy improvisation in which therapist and client are flowing together, sharing musical impulses with uncanny sensitivity and responsiveness towards one another, then we can say that both partners organise themselves coherently, in an intersubjective context. The partners 'know' one another intimately, in a dynamic, non-referential, motivational sense. Their interaction is highly synchronous in that they meet, match and reflect aspects of one another, attuning to one another through spontaneous music-making of great fluidity and flexibility.

I conclude this discussion by addressing various aspects to do with Dynamic Form. These various aspects are not necessarily presents coherently, or synchronously, but may be thought of as other directions for thinking about music therapy improvisation.

Beyond Meeting and Matching: Sketching the Limits

Growing towards

In terms of the therapeutic aspect of music therapy, it is not always helpful to the client for the therapist to match and meet the client's musical acts: in order that the client might grow into a fuller experience of him or herself, and in order that he or she might begin to explore the full potential of his or her Dynamic Form, the therapist may need occasionally to mis-match, thereby offering something new.

For example, in work with a man who suffered from Huntington's disease (described in more detail later in this chapter), the therapist not only meets the client's jerky, rhythmic movements, but also provides a stable base that is 'out of sync' with the client. This mis-matching alerts the client to potential new directions in the music, and in himself.

However, the therapist's mis-matching needs to be congruent with the music being played. Music that differs too strongly – or that is too mis-matched – results in the client not responding to or rejecting the therapist's offer. This act of rejection, which suggests that the person has a strong enough sense of self *not* simply to comply with all of the therapist's clinical 'requests', often falls under the label of 'resistiveness'. For example, the client might stop playing, begin talking, or ignore the therapist's changes and continue with his or her own music. Here, clearly, the therapist's clinical intervention is inappropriate in the first instance. As music therapists, we need to ensure that we too are part of the equation when suggesting that the client is 'resistive'. Are *we*, in fact, 'in tune'?

This is a parallel communicative dynamic to infants whose mothers are asked to hold 'blank faces' with their infants, who then become distressed and distracted as a result. Here the mother's mis-matching of her infant's states is 'unnatural' and incongruent with the infant's acts. This the infant senses, and becomes distressed, ceasing to feel 'met' by the mother, and eventually losing interest in the interaction (Murray 1992; Murray and Stein 1991).

Thinking neurologically

How else can the improvisation be 'read'? Is clinical improvisation only about relationship? Can it be about eliciting a profile of the client? If so, what kind of profile? If what is needed is a neurological assessment or profile, it seems rather confusing to engage in an interactive and highly dynamic clinical improvisation simply in order to glean information about the client's capacity to, for example, co-ordinate his or her physical acts. Indeed, here the interactive nature of the act may well confuse the information sought. The eliciting of a neurological profile about a client is perhaps best left to specialists: we can leave this to contexts that ask persons to reproduce sounds, imitate, extend and invert melodies, much in the same way as Alexander Luria's psychoneurological investigations through music (Christensen 1974) or in terms of the traditional aural tests that musicians undergo as part of their training. We do not need an interactive context in order to elicit this information but, at the same time, where there is a neurological dysfunction or a physical trauma or injury, it may be that in addressing the *emotional* life of the patient through music therapy, the patient becomes motivated, because of the positive feelings generated in the improvisation, to extend, alter and stabilise his or her movements. In this sense we cannot separate the emotional components to our physical and neurological acts (Magee 1995).

Catharsis

It is also limiting to think of clinical improvisation purely as a cathartic exercise, in which energy is 'ejected' through musical acts, thus giving relief to the person. This may be part of what occurs, but it happens within a broader palette. I did, however, once have a one-off music therapy session with a middle-aged woman, at her request. Within moments of beginning to play the cymbal she began to weep, and this soon escalated into a full-blown expression of forceful cries, hard and deafening beating on the cymbal, hammering of fists on the wall, all of which I contained, as best as I could, at the piano, attempting to meet and match the energy, the shape and the timing of her howls. After what felt like a very long and loud time, her cries began to subside, and she stopped rather suddenly, picked up her handbag, thanked me perfunctorily and left the room. I never saw her again, but learnt afterwards that she had requested music therapy through her GP, since previous sessions with another music therapist had helped her to 'let rip'. The session was undoubtedly cathartic for her (and it left me feeling totally wrung out), but it was not especially interactive: she did what she needed to 'be allowed' to do, in a context that suited her – but our engagement was rather limited. Esme Towse (1991) makes the same point in her description of a client who 'let rip' while she, the therapist, was out of the room: the client did not seem to need the therapist's physical presence during this event.

Ways of being

The improvisation offers an opportunity to re-create 'ways of being' in the world, to enable therapist and client to experience how it feels to be in the world within an environment that is not threatening, abusive or exploitative; within an environment that has potential for playing, for fun, for abandonment and for personal growth, in whatever dimension that growth needs to take place. Part of this personal growth may involve the physical experience of the stabilising of movement for a jerky, uncoordinated, spasmodic person, because this enables them to extend their experience of sharing with another person; it may be developing intentionality in vocal sounds; it may be coming to accept that one's disease will not go away; it may be an opportunity to express difficult or taboo feelings; it may be about freeing oneself from inhibiting constraints imposed by families or society – and so on.

People suffering from a whole range of disabilities manifest distortions in aspects of verbal as well as non-verbal communication. Some speech disturbances have purely 'musical' or prosodic dysfunctions, while remaining semantically intact. Some disabilities are manifested in disturbed timing of movements, speech, gestures – here we can think of someone suffering from Huntington's disease, someone who has had a stroke or a brain injury or someone who is severely depressed, while the 'aphasias' refer to a disturbance in speech semantics, rather than prosody. For example, people who suffer from a psychotic illness may jumble up their words, as in 'word salad', or use language extremely floridly; people who suffer from autistic features also show idiosyncratic speech. There may even be a total absence of speech, as in the case of someone with a profound mental handicap, a severe stroke or severe brain injury.

In many of these instances, where words are unreliable or altogether absent, we rely on non-verbal cues in order to share meaning and intentions. Bronwen Burford's work (1988) has shown that non-verbal intimate interactions between carers and profoundly handicapped people have elements of cyclical patterns and rhythmicity that have a stable tempo base, despite the handicapped people's gross, as well as fine, motor handicaps. Here, although words are absent, and socially prescribed rituals and behaviours have not been 'learnt', a high level of intimacy is possible between carers and persons. This is akin to the intimacy of mothers and new-born infants.

Dysfunctions of timing, intensity, shape and motion may be portrayed in music therapy improvisation, where the therapist meets the person, not in a 'musically satisfying' way (e.g., playing in regular tempo, with a musical fluctuation of intensity, and so on), but adapting her playing in order to reflect, meet and match the person, and inviting them, in their idiosyncratic, mis-timed and limited way, to be part of an improvisation that 'fits' them.

I once worked with a middle-aged man who had been a highly successful businessman and had been diagnosed as suffering from Huntington's disease. His speech was slurred but semantically intact, his gait was unsteady, but he was still able to ascend and descend stairs, although he could no longer drive. Unsurprisingly, he was depressed and despairing about his life in a world that was rapidly becoming elusive to his asynchronous movements. In our jointly created, spontaneous musical improvisations, there was a jerkiness of rhythm and pulse, an unpredictability that took some getting used to: his playing would catch me off guard, so to speak, and at first my own pulse and tempo used to miss his, thus, no doubt, reinforcing his experience of 'being missed' or being unattuned to. Gradually I became aware that a strong triple metre enabled him to steady himself and settle into something akin to the periodicity which had become so distorted because of his illness. I began to set a strong metrical pulse with strong, warm harmonic textures that were Schumannesque in colour. This metre I would hold, so that he could organise himself and move towards it. My holding of the metred pulse while he adjusted his own playing laboriously (and often pouring with perspiration) took some discipline on my part: it was extremely uncomfortable to be 'out of synchrony' with him, as well as, at times, to experience his physical contortions. However, the stable musical base, as well as 'waiting' for him while in motion (so that he did not experience the world as waiting in that 'dead' or 'static' sense: the music was moving *and* waiting at the same time) provided him with a simple and accessible invariant to join. He expressed enormous satisfaction and emotional release at the music we made together. I believe that by providing him with an experience of being met and matched, and of his having to meet and match me, within his physical capacities in his increasingly blurred and unsteady world, music therapy was providing a dignified emotional intimacy that was slipping away from him. This, of course, had nothing to do with words. Wendy Magee has described the contrast between 'Caroline', who suffered from Huntington's disease, when she was part of a music group and showed animation and pleasure in her music-making, and the Caroline who tended to sit still, interact very little and whose severely impaired speech and impaired awareness of others left her isolated and withdrawn (Magee 1995).

There is a direct reciprocity between our internal states, our external expression of these, whether verbal or not, and the feedback we receive from a world that experiences us as difficult to attune to, because of, e.g., odd, jerky movements and gestures and unclear speech. This is surely one of the causes of the profound depression that accompanies patients' rehabilitation from strokes. Music improvisation can be created on the spot in such a way as to attune to the patient's vitality affects, of swooping, jerking, bursting, being drawn out, being thick and muddy, or whatever, and the isolated person can feel met and 'shared with'. Here is a world that is 'good enough' in the Winnicottian sense, and here is a world that provides an intersubjective experience. This intimate sharing of internal states between therapist and patient is demanding and enriching to both partners, in the same way that mothers are in love with their babies – this knowing intimately of another person is a state that is akin to love. And certainly therapists have strong feelings about their clients, even negative feelings: this is the stuff of intimate relationships that impinge as much on the therapists as on the clients. Hence the need for stable and secure 'therapeutic boundaries' in order to 'contain' the music therapy sessions, as we shall see in the next section.

In the more subtle dysfunctions of mood or affect, i.e. dysfunctions that have no clear-cut clinical basis or physical component, the affective states are portrayed far more subtly through Dynamic Form. Here it is the *shifts* of relating and non-relating, of who takes the initiative and how and when, of the quality of the responsiveness, that are highlighted through musical utterances. These may be highly flexible and smooth, and display a capacity to tolerate fragmentation, and a confidence to venture towards new and daring musical territory. Without wishing to insist on 'pathological' aspects of clinical improvisation, in highly fluid and flexible improvisations where there is a strong sense of relationship between therapist and client, then the therapist may need to reflect on 'what is missing' – what is 'not there'. For instance, somewhere along the jointly created spectrum of expressive, interactive flexibility there may be a block or a ceiling that feels out of balance with the total inter-personal musical picture. Here I can think of a (neurologically intact) young man whose improvisations displayed a fairly static level of intensity: in terms of vitality affects, he seemed unable to 'swoosh' or 'swoop', but remained stuck somewhere on that range of intensity. This was at odds with his capacity for rhythmic complexity, melodic variety, and so on, and left me somewhat puzzled. In talking about the improvisation afterwards, he himself made the connection between this intermusical experience in music therapy and his need to be in control of his life: he felt that he could not allow himself to 'let go', because of fears that all would fall apart if he were to do so. Now this is hardly a clinical state, nor is it a condition that might be labelled 'pathological' in the formal sense of the word. And yet something in our improvisation was not quite complete – it remained a niggle, and this was one of the areas that we worked with, together. In working with a young woman whose freedom of expression resulted in free and very exciting Dynamic Form, I had a clinical niggle that I could not quite put my finger on. It was in my clinical supervision sessions that I was helped to 'hear' what was missing: the music was complex, free, subtly shifting and flexible, and what was lacking was simplicity. The more I reflected on this absence, the more aware I became of this young adult's avoidance of contact that was direct and simple, and my own difficulty in offering this, becoming constantly seduced by her complex and beguiling music. Here we are approaching concepts such as transference and counter-transference, which I have chosen purposely to leave out of this discussion on Dynamic Form.

There is a whole spectrum of music therapy work that cannot be limited to the concept of Dynamic Form. Here I am thinking especially of work with self-referred adults, people who choose to come to music therapy in order to explore emotional and relational aspects of their lives. In this instance, the various meanings of the improvisations need to be negotiated between therapist and client. For example, the improvisation may have direct refer-ential meaning for the client.; it may reflect, create, and extend mood states, or recreate relational scenarios in the client's life. To think of this kind of work only in terms of Dynamic Form is limiting. The range, complexities and subtleties of non-musical meaning need eliciting – often verbally, and here Dynamic Form adds – and indeed, may generate – significance to the discussion. This area of meaning extends towards the arena of psychody-namic thought, which will be explored in the next section.

In Conclusion

The concept of Dynamic Form crystallises why music makes therapeutic sense. By understanding the dual nature of Dynamic Form, we can draw multi-faceted meaning from the jointly created musical form. The musical panorama becomes a complex and multi-faceted one, which does not pretend to be coherent or entirely logical: indeed, as Marion Milner (1957) states, we need to resist the temptation to make things 'fit' into order and logic. By doing so we risk diminishing its shades of meaning.

At the same time, it is not convincing to suppose that the meaning of the music is simply itself, and I strongly refute the stance that to understand the music musically, so to speak, is to absorb fully the therapeutic meaning of 'musically', but my guess is that this limitation of meaning impinges – albeit subtly – on the quality of the relationship and on the depth of the work. At the same time, however, there may be too much meaning and no musical substance – a flimsy musical experience may generate a multitude of meanings which remain within the therapist's head. I am not sure that this is helpful to the client. The meaning may of course be discussed and shared verbally, but then I wonder whether, in this instance, we need music at all.

The next section of this book adds to the complexity of the therapeutic meeting, by drawing from psychodynamic theory in order to address what happens 'around' the improvisation.

PART III

CHAPTER 10

Meaning in Relationship
A View from Psychodynamic Theory

Clinical improvisation defines itself in the relationship that develops between therapist and client, and the meaning elicited in the relationship is meaning that belongs to both the therapist and client. Both partners are a part of what happens in the improvisation. When detaching the meaning from the actual live experience of music therapy, and exploring the meaning as a separate phenomenon, it seems critical to retain the dynamism of the relationship between the therapist and client – a portrayal of only the client, that excludes the therapist, seems incomplete. The chapters in this section focus on the relationship: on what it might mean, on its various aspects and how we might understand them.

Ways of Seeing
Much of psychodynamic theory explores meaning as rooted in, and generating from, the relationship between therapist and client, and it is from this discourse that I now draw in order to broaden and enrich this exploration of 'the meaning between'. As stated earlier, the verbal basis for psychodynamic psychotherapy is not a convincing reason not to draw from this literature – and, in any case, psychotherapy is based on much more than 'words', in the same way that music therapy is about much more than 'music'.

Before delving into 'meaning in relationship', it seems important to clarify that not all music therapists emphasise the importance of the relationship between the therapist and the client in their work. Some may work in the 'medical model', where the emphasis may be on diagnosing and 'treating' the client/patient; some may use a behavioural or a cognitive approach, emphasising, rather, the client's response to the music and/or to the therapist. This orientation towards the client may be seen as being 'profile-oriented', where the therapist attempts to create a picture of the client's state and how the client might be treated according to that profile. In this section, the therapeutic relationship is considered to be central to the music therapy work: the relationship *is* the therapeutic event, and this event is created, together and concurrently, by therapist and client.

What also needs some thought is that there is a wide range of descriptions, portrayals, assessment and 'truths' within the profession, and before delving into psychodynamic theory it may be useful to consider where this 'way of seeing' is appropriate and where it is not. It may be helpful, here, to separate the music therapy act from the way that this act is understood, explained, described and portrayed – and theorised about. In order to gain some clarity about various positions, I treat them as mutually exclusive – which is, of course, rather artificial.

At one end of the spectrum, we might understand the clinical work as being 'purely musical'. Here the music itself is considered to be inherently therapeutic, and the clinical event may be portrayed through *musical* terms leaving the music to 'speak for itself'. Within this position, therapists might say that the very strength of music therapy is the music, and this does not need words indeed, words might get in the way of the intimacy and directness of the relationship. Where music therapists work with clients who, in any case, do not speak or have no access to verbal language, this position is a powerful one.

A bit further along this spectrum is the position that although the therapy happens through the music – through clinical use of music – its meaning is more than just musical. However, this meaning can 'look after itself', and does not need to be delved into – and certainly not through words. A little further along is the position of the 'behavioural' or 'cognitive' music therapist, who assigns behavioural or cognitive meaning to the music therapy act, using this language in order to describe the event. The 'musical' language may be completely ignored and replaced by neurological, physiologi-cal,and/or behavioural terms.

At another point on the spectrum is the position that music is inherently therapeutic, that the therapist and client do not necessarily need to talk about it (and, indeed, the client may not be able to talk), but the therapist needs to absorb the full, complex, multi-faceted meaning of the event, which under-standing will inform the therapeutic act, embodied through the jointly created improvisation.

Further along our imaginary spectrum is the position that the musical event generates meaning that needs to be talked about, and unless this meaning is talked about, then the therapeutic event remains incomplete, and the client is unable to bring the event into his or her consciousness.

I now want to frame these positions within the realm of psychodynamic thinking (Figure 10.1). It seems that we can divide the above positions into two camps, rather crudely identified as this: those music therapists whose work 'means' according to the psychodynamic frame of reference, and those whose work does not. In each of these camps, music therapists might use only music, or might use words and music. However, what distinguishes the one from the other is that each camp *thinks* about the work in a certain way. It is the psychodynamic 'set of meanings' that is explored in the next chapters. The other camp, whose work does not 'mean' psychodynamically, may work exclusively through the music – and say, therefore, that the meaning is exclusively musical; or they may use both words and music, but these are not used within a psychodynamic frame of reference.

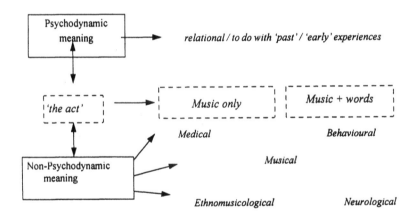

Figure 10.1 The relationship between the act and its meaning

Thus it is not the presence or absence of words that defines an approach as being psychodynamically informed or not, as is sometimes, rather confusingly, stated in the argument for and against the use of words in music therapy (see Figure 10.2). Rather it is the way that the practice is thought about – is meant – that distinguishes a psychodynamic from a non-psychodynamic approach. Moreover, some clinical work carried out under the 'non-psychodynamic' label may, in fact, be very close to psychodynamic work, but may not be using this discourse to describe itself. The next chapters, while exploring psychodynamic thinking in music therapy, will also attempt to bear in mind the fact that this is not the only way of portraying the work.

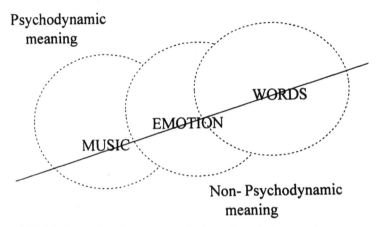

Figure 10.2 Music, words and emotion may be 'meant' psychodynamically or non-psychodynamically, in music therapy

Before beginning this exploration, I want to clarify some of the terms used in the following chapters.

Despite their distinctions, delete in theory and in practice, I choose here not to treat psychoanalysis, psychoanalytically informed psychotherapy, and psychotherapy, as discrete categories. Rather I see them as moving along a spectrum that takes into account, with varying degrees of intensity and interlinking, the client's present, the influences of the past on the present, and the relationship between therapist and client as re-creating aspects of past relationships. I do, however, choose to draw the line to exclude counselling, which I see as having to do essentially with the client's present life context, and therefore being less relevant here. In the remainder of the chapter, the words 'analyst' and 'therapist' are used interchangeably, as are 'analytic' and 'therapeutic', with no apology to the more fundamentalist-inclined practitioners. I also use the terms 'clients' and 'patients' interchangeably, as an acknowledgement that many music therapists work in medical settings, where they see patients, and that the term 'client' refers to one who engages the professional services of another.

Boundaries, Frames and Spaces

Quite apart from the 'surface' boundaries that therapists of all persuasions set in terms of duration of sessions, days and times of sessions, the use of premises for sessions, contracts with clients in terms of payments and, in some cases, duration of treatment, there are other boundaries that emerge in therapy. These contain spaces created by both therapist and client in therapy. Donald Winnicott (1971) talks about therapy taking place within a 'space between' two people – therapist and client – and the quality of what this space symbolises is clarified for me by the ever-inspiring Patrick Casement (1985, 1988). Casement describes the space in therapy as being framed, and this framing separates it from the world outside. The space protects the patient from external intrusions and from the claims that people make upon one another in everyday interactions. This protection of the space enables a particular way of relating to emerge between therapist and patient: one that enables the bringing into focus of the patient's past and the way that it spills into the present. The analyst, too, needs to be alert to keeping the space 'pure' or 'sacred', and needs to attend to, and check, his or her own potential for interfering and intruding into the space. One of the main functions of the therapeutic space is to enable the client to feel safe enough within it to risk feeling unsafe. The space enables intimacy to develop between therapist and client, and this intimacy contains its own internal spaciousness.

Defining the space

The therapeutic space can be thought of as a twilight zone, where a more diffuse light allows a particular way of seeing and listening to both the inner and the outer world, one that is often trivialised and minimised in the glare of daily life.

Therapeutic space is pertinent for music therapists. One of the questions for music therapists is how we define the therapeutic space. Is the space only the actual musical improvisation, in other words, is it the music that distinguishes between what is framed (the music) and what is not framed, or does the therapeutic space include both words and music? If the space includes non-musical events – for example, words – then we ask whether the 'music space' is a separate space to the 'non-music space', or whether, as Elaine Streeter (1995) puts it, the music and the non-music are part of the totality of experience between therapist and client.

In writing about frames in art therapy contexts, Marion Milner (1957) suggests that frames of paintings distinguish between life and symbol. When there is a frame, she says, it serves to indicate that what is inside it has to be interpreted in a different way to what is outside it: a frame can be seen as the boundary between what is to be taken symbolically and what is taken literally. In music therapy, do we understand frames as distinguishing between clinical improvisation and 'pure' music improvisation; between music and words; between different aspects within the therapeutic space? Can we listen to what is within the musical frame in one way and listen to what is outside it another way? Do we say, for example, that what is outside the music frame and is in a different 'mode' needs a different conceptual framework? Can we blur the frames and listen and see the totality?

The meeting place

This way of thinking about frames highlights events that have already been 'exteriorised', embodied in music, words, silences and gestures, by the therapist and client. The frames allow these events to be available to complex meanings and interpretations by therapist and client.

There is another kind of frame or boundary, however, and this concerns the meeting point between inner images and their outer realities. The inner image – which we can think of in terms of being the pre-image or the unsounded sound – rests within, in the heart of the self, so to speak, and in this sense it is within a frame. This inner imagine may not find complete expression in the sounded act (or in the painting), and here we might imagine the frame as holding back something of the image, preventing it from being fully realised. Conversely, we might also think of the exterior reality as being framed, and this exterior frame as including some of the inner qualities, and leaving them behind. If we frame a certain aspect of the therapy experience as being the only true space – the space that contains the embodiment of the inner image, then it seems that we narrow the possibilities for inviting and apprehending a more complete image – and for holding in mind aspects of the images that are not being sounded.

But what about creating the musical space in the first place? Earlier we touched on the discomfort that many high-functioning, non-impaired adults express about playing music. Many people in industrial and post-industrial societies live with personal legacies of being told that they are 'unmusical'. They feel uncomfortable about the idea of music therapy, supposing that it should be left to skilled musicians who have had musical training. The music therapist's first task is, then, to guide the client away from 'conventionally coded' music, towards making spontaneous sounds-of-the-self, and not judging the sounds that they create by the standards of tunes they know and like or by preconceived standards of what is and is not music (Ansdell 1995; Pavlicevic 1987, 1995b; Roberts 1996). Here, it seems, the therapist needs to support the client's cautious and tentative creating of the frame, if the frame is 'just musical'. Inevitably the question of coercion emerges: do we, as music therapists, coerce clients into making music? Is there a sense – albeit subtle – in which we expect clients to 'play our tune'? This issue is somewhat addressed by seeing the entire session as being framed, and the client's reluctance and discomfort with playing is part of the therapeutic process and is included in the therapeutic frame.

At the same time, however, an ease and comfort with playing music does not simplify the concept of framing – and, in my experience, this may often result in an 'inauthentic' musical boundary being defined. My experience of living in a culture that has managed to maintain and sustain a significant (although intangible) pre-industrial, indigenous culture, is that its members experience little musical inhibitions. The social musicianship of sub-Saharan Africa is legendary (Blacking 1973) and, in my experience, this carries its own difficulties with regard to music therapy. My experience of working with groups of black South Africans is that the group dives into the 'music' mode that is familiar: highly ritualised and socially ubiquitous. This musical frame often feels out of focus: in my (First World therapy) mind, the shift needs to be made from 'social' music, defined over centuries of ritual, to 'clinical' music that emerges from how the group is in the moment.

The 'social' music, of course, conveys something about the group dynamic. Nevertheless, the music's framework, style and idiom, as well as its symbolic and social meanings, may detract from bringing the group's dynamic into a sharper focus. In instances such as these, the social nuances of the group ensure that the space has already been defined swiftly and tightly by the group. This space often excludes me instantly because it is a culturally defined space. Nothing about the music (or the language) is negotiated between us, nor is the meaning of a song accessible to me. When I was less familiar with local cultural norms, I frequently reacted negatively to what felt like a sealed space that was displayed with such cheerful exclusiveness. Moreover, the cultural norms in South Africa can be excruciatingly difficult to read in a society which has compromised its indigenous identity in the interests of survival in a colonial context.

This colonisation presents further complexities: how can I, as the group facilitator, use that very experience to bring to the group's attention how we define exclusive space that excludes rather than invites others – without colonising the group with Western ideas about group dynamics? This highlights the need for the therapeutic frame to be negotiated between therapist and client, rather than being simply imposed and designed by the therapist. The (anxious, unmusical, self-referred adult) client, for a start, may not even want to play at all. And then what?

Multiplying the space

In conclusion, we need, perhaps, to consider the therapeutic space in another way. Rather than seeing it as one space with various facets, some more prominent, at times, than others, we can also consider a multi-levelled space, made up of various screens (Figure 10.3) between and through which we constantly shift. Thus we can think of a music screen in which we relate musically; another in which we relate verbally; a screen in which we think in musical concepts; one through which we listen and experience the musical act; one in which verbal thinking dominates the way that we listen to both the verbal and the musical; one screen in which our thinking is psychotherapeutic; one in which musical compositional rules prevail, and so on. We can then see ourselves as switching between screens, both during and after the sessions.[1]

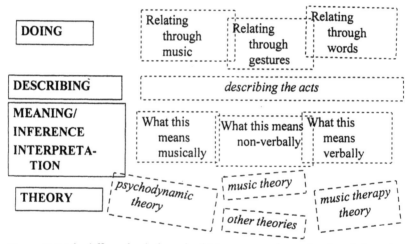

Figure 10.3 The different levels through which we may understand and explain sessions

Whatever and however as music therapists we conceptualise therapeutic boundaries and spaces, it seems to me that these need to be fluid and courageous; they need to drift towards and beyond, as well as within, the music improvisation. Our minds, as music therapists, need to dare to break the 'rules' if we are to come anywhere near truly 'being with' the client.

---

1   The idea of screens through which we look at sessions came during a conversation with Sandra Brown at the Nordoff–Robbins International MT Symposium, 1995 in London. I had been thinking of vertical screens of increasing depth, rather like peering into the depths of the sea, and she suggested that they might be seen as one in front of, and behind, the other.

CHAPTER 11

Playing with Winnicott's Reality[1]

Where Does Music Therapy Happen?

Music therapists, like most expressive arts therapists, love Winnicott. I include myself in the many who quote Winnicott with phrases such as, 'therapy takes place in the potential space between therapist and client', therapy has to do with 'play' and 'not-play', therapy has to do with the therapist being 'good enough', the therapist 'holding', music being the 'intermediary' field, music as 'transitional phenomena' – and so on.

But why, particularly, Winnicott? Why not Klein, Guntrip, Kohut, Jung, Adler, Freud, *et al.*? Is it that his language is graphic, a mixture of concrete and artistic; that his images are accessible; that he focuses on 'play' and 'creativity', both of which are close to arts therapists' belief systems; that his concepts clarify something about the arts therapies? Here I expand on earlier ideas (Pavlicevic 1991, 1995a) of how and why music therapy thinking is enriched by some of his more accessible concepts, in the context of music therapy: those of 'creativity' of 'autonomy' and of 'playing'.

Creativity and Autonomy

Primary creativity

Winnicott (1971, 1988, 1990) understands creativity as having to do with how we fit in with the world and its details, and the degree with which we can be both part of, and separate from, the world and its objects. He approaches the concept of primary creativity from the baby's first moments after birth, suggesting that the baby has something to contribute to the first interaction with the world – e.g. the first feed. He suggests that primary creativity is distinguishable, not so much by the originality of the production

---

1   I am grateful to Sandra Brown for her comments and suggestions for this and the following two chapters.

(i.e., creating something anew) as by the individual's sense of reality of the experience as growing out of, and becoming distinct from, illusion. Winnicott speaks of the infant's ego 'building up strength' towards a state when id-demands are felt as part of the self, and not environmental. Each individual has the potential to create the world anew, a task that begins, 'at least as early as at the time of birth and of the theoretical first feed' (1988, p.110). What and how the infant creates depends largely on the mother's capacity to make creative adaptation to the infant's needs, but the creativity needs to be present in the infant in the first place. Winnicott suggests, also, that the issues of primary creativity persist for as long as the person is alive – primary creativity is not confined to the dependent state of infancy.

If we think of creativity in these terms, then the expression of the creative impulse is related to our capacity to perceive the world objectively: this means that we can distinguish between what is 'real' and what is 'illusion'. At the same time, however, we have the capacity to conceive the world subjectively – i.e. our capacity to create the world ourselves, to create our own version of the world. These two interplay with one another constantly, throughout our lives. The capacity to hold both means that we need to be strong enough and confident enough to distinguish the boundary between ourselves and the 'outer' world (i.e., what is 'me' and what is 'not me') and to acknowledge the constantly shifting balance between our inner world and the outer world. We relate to the world of objects 'out there', but also through internalising the world, knowing it from the 'inside', in other words we need to be able to create it within, for ourselves.

Autonomy

In order to distinguish between the inner and outer world, we need a sufficiently developed sense of 'authentic' autonomy, enabling us, as a unique person, to image and create subjectively and to be confident in the authenticity of our images. We need to know that the world of objects is not going to 'swallow us up', nor is it going to invade us and take over our inner world.

The absence of authentic autonomy may be described as our incapacity to shift between our inner and outer world. At one extreme, we may be separated from the external world of objects, which we may experience as distant and as having a dream-like quality. Here our autonomy is false, in the sense that we need to 'seal off' the external world in order to experience autonomy within our inner world. This world is experienced as falsely safe: we feel autonomous since we need to feel that we have total control over the world. In extreme cases, this is the realm of the person who has a psychotic illness: delusions and hallucinations can be seen as the person existing essentially in their inner world, which needs to remain as sealed and separate as possible from the outer world. The latter is perceived as threatening, frightening and capable of overwhelming the person, and violating this false sense of autonomy.

At the other extreme, we may be seen as existing mostly in the external world of objects, and as being out of touch with our internal life. The autonomy experienced here is also false: by being out of touch with our inner world and its less predictable movements, we experience a false sense of security. From this position, the world of (internal) objects appears easy to organise and manipulate. We may also remain in the 'outer' world because, conversely, it is unsafe and too unpredictable to allow us respite from it. My own experience of this syndrome on a macro social scale was while living in South Africa between 1991 and 1994. The years leading up to the momentous elections in April 1994 were characterised by extreme tension and violence in the country as a whole. Within this climate of uncertainty, it was difficult to be in touch with one's inner world: events 'out there' were moving too quickly, and were extremely powerful in the anxiety that they provoked. One dared not relieve one's 'outer' vigilance and turn 'inwards', in case something critical happened during one's absence, so to speak. This caused enormous stress within all of us living there at the time, and it was this that prompted my setting up creative improvisation groups with adults, as a forum for 'playing' – literally allowing ourselves time and space with our inner lives (Pavlicevic 1994, 1995b, 1995c).

Playing in the world
According to Winnicott, it is through play that we acquire a sustained sense of subjectivity and agency in the world – a subjectivity with a sense of coherence, a sense of history and a sense of continuity. It is through playing, as infants, with our mothers and later with transitional objects, that we acquire a sense of contrast between our inner world and the actual/external reality. The security generated by a transitional object that is always available (even when the mother is increasingly less available), helps us to gain a sense of the world that is sustained – the world, symbolised by the transitional object, will not disappear. Through playing we acquire a sense of that which is and that which is not, that which may be, that which ought to be, that which could be and that which will be. Play, according to Winnicott, takes place somewhere in the vast intermediate area between reality that is absolute, and fantasy. Playing enables us to bridge the gap between what is 'there' and what is 'not there' – we can pretend that the world is 'there' even when it is

not; we can 'try out' different ways of being in and with the world. Play leads us towards authentic autonomy.

According to Winnicott, mental illness and disturbances in emotional life may be described as the absence of authentic autonomy or as an incapacity to tolerate uncertainty. Illness, in this sense, can be seen as the degree to which primary creativity is hidden: the individual does not have a sufficiently cohered and developed sense of self to be able to make sense of the world, to test and play with different boundaries between the self and other, or to create and image the world within. There is a difficulty or collapsed capacity to distinguish between what is illusory and what is real. We know that children who have no coherent sense of self, as a result of psychic trauma, cannot play. They lack the sense of a sufficiently integrated sense of the 'I', to have any sense of subjective agency that is necessary for play. Illness may be described as the absence of authentic autonomy, i.e. a confusion as to whether one's self begins and the outer world ends.

Contrary to popular belief, the link between mental illness and creativity is inexact: although several artists of great stature suffered from 'mental illnesses' at one or other time, Anthony Storr (1972) explains that during the actual episodes of illness the creative output stops. He suggests, rather, that the reason why artistic people are 'off-beat' and slightly 'odd' is because they are more in touch with what he calls 'their pathology' (which I take to mean the inner world and all its chaos and unreasonableness), and more able to straddle the inner and outer realities and tolerate the ambiguities therein. In other words, artistic people could be said to have more ego strength and are able to tolerate the uncertainty of straddling the inner and outer world.

Playing in Music Therapy

Winnicott's (1971) understanding of playing is a useful analogy for extending our understanding of clinical improvisation. In playing within the potential space between itself and the mother, the baby develops the capacity for receiving ideas (or objects) introduced by another. This paves the way for further playing together in a relationship: one that begins, increasingly, to be able to tolerate the inclusion of 'objects'. The baby's use of the potential space of communication is related to his confidence and trust in the adaptability and dependability of the environment provided by the (m)other. Where there is mistrust and fear of the environment, the creative potential of the potential space is threatening and frightening, since it is felt that it may disappear or disintegrate. Where the potential space can be filled confidently with the products of the baby's imagination, it offers the opportunity to shape and reshape images. Thus playing takes place neither in the inner world nor in the outer world, but in the potential space between mother and infant. Play offers the possibility of testing the fluidity of boundaries between our inner and outer world, by the very act of testing the boundaries between ourselves and others.

In a similar way, when a music therapist and patient are able to create a shared musical space between them, within which both express themselves by playing, then an intimate and dynamic intersubjective relationship is possible. For this to happen, the therapist needs to enable the patient to express him or herself through the music (Pavlicevic 1991). Clinical improvisation – which happens between therapist and client – embodies the joint creation of a mutually accessible and convenient musical space. This musical space exists between therapist and client: it is part of 'me' and 'not me', for each of the partners, and is also 'there' and 'not there' in the sense of being, and also not being, 'the world'. The act of the therapist and client together creating the musical space is an act of playing in the Winnicottian sense: the client is invited, through the simple act of, say, beating a drum, to 'have a say' in creating a play-full space. The therapist, by listening to the quality of the drumbeat (its tempo, dynamic, timbre, degree of organisation, etc.) acknowledges the client as stating, through the beating, 'this is who and how I am, now, and how I can be with you'. By musically matching the qualities of the client's beating through improvising in a way that meets the client's rhythm, dynamic, timbre, tempo, rhythmic forms, the therapist is stating, 'I acknowledge who and how you are'. Together, through a highly spontaneous interchange of musical phrases and rhythmic patterns, the therapist and client negotiate how the musical space is to be used between them, while at the same time continuing to create and extend it. One of the therapist's first clinical tasks may be of inviting the client(s) to play with another person – the therapist – in order that their joint dynamic form can be sounded.

As we have seen, clinical improvisation reveals that people with emotional difficulties are less able to organise their musical utterances: even a basic beat or regular pulse may not be possible, and this renders a shared or two-way interaction difficult to establish. The joint clinical improvisations may reveal dynamic forms which are fragmented, inflexible or incoherent to the therapist, who then has great difficulty in mutually creating a musical play-full space with the client. This we can understand as an embodiment of a fragmented sense of self, and of confusion as to where the boundaries between the inner and outer word lie. In severe instances the therapist's work is far more that of a 'care-taker': the therapist may have to create music 'for' rather than 'with' the client, while acknowledging, through her music (and it is *her* music, at this point, rather than *their* music) the client's lack of coherence. For example, when the client's playing is extremely fragmented, with no predictability of, say, rhythmic form or pulse, the therapist may 'join in' the fragmentation, holding it up to the client as a 'mirror'. This enables the client to hear him or herself within an accepting environment: the music is in no way judging or even commenting on the fragmentation, but rather the therapist, through reflecting the client's music, is 'being with' the client. No matter how confusing and lacking in 'authentic autonomy', and no matter how limited the ground for 'playing' , the client has a direct experience (which may well bypass perception and cognition and conscious thought), that his or her world is shareable with another.

However, my clinical experience of work with persons suffering from chronic schizophrenia is that for the 'fragmented' client to hear that degree of fragmentation reflected can be extremely distressing, and may, indeed, add to the client's sense of a confusing and confused boundary between the 'self' and the 'other', as well as between the 'inner' and the 'outer' world. In contrast, my experience of offering a structured – possibly highly structured – musical environment that manages to catch something of the client's quality, often provides the client with a feeling of being met and contained: his or her fragmentation and disorder can resonate with something more ordered – and this order is recognisable, for it contains something of the client in it.

I once worked with – played with – a young man whose music can only be described as ongoing chaos. His beats had no order, predictability or underlying periodicity – and I spent a lot of time pondering what on earth to do, musically, with what he was offering me. Around our third session I stumbled into a very slow, smooth, utterly laid-back swing. This music had endlessly elastic spaces between the beats, which at first seemed rather incongruent with his tight, disorganised 'noise', for that was how it sounded to me. And yet I had an immediate sense that this music was 'right' for us. It was loose enough to tolerate endless and chaotic busy-ness in between the beats, while at the same time being structured enough to hold us both – for I, too, without any doubt, needed holding. In work such as this, we could say that 'playing', in the Winnicottian sense, is limited: the avenues for stating, extending, trying out new boundaries and venturing towards more unusual horizons seem shorter, and much of the work is in containing, holding, sustaining the person's sense of coherence: that they are one person and they have a beginning and an end. This resonates with Anne Alvarez' (1992) thoughts that the client with a fragmented sense of self needs to be given a vocabulary with which to play, i.e. with which to develop a sense of self that is coherent enough to be able to begin being an agent in the world.

Thus in music therapy, it is the 'emotional' creativity – or the individual's capacity for autonomy – rather than 'artistic' creativity, that is being tapped in improvisation, despite the 'artistic' or 'aesthetic' medium being used. This is because the ingredients or elements of music reveal this intra- and inter-psychic dynamic directly, without referential or semantic meaning to confuse or distract from it.

Artistic Creativity and Primary Creativity

The concept of primary creativity enhances and extends our understanding of creativity, which has become typically associated with 'art'. In thinking about Winnicott's primary creativity, we see that creativity can have to do, quite simply, with 'being alive' – with being in, and engaging with, the world. This may have little to do with being an 'artist'.

The potential for confusing artistic creativity and emotional creativity is exacerbated in music therapy (and, indeed, in any art therapy), which uses a medium that is traditionally the sphere of artistic creativity, and has a separate, richly established tradition of what constitutes 'creative' or 'uncreative' (i.e. value judgements about good and bad music). As arts therapists, we need to be clear about the distinction between creativity that has to do with a work of art – or 'purely' artistic creativity – and creativity that has to do with emotional creativity, or our emotional life. As arts therapists we tap the emotional creativity of a person, rather than their artistic creativity, through the medium that is traditionally associated with artistic creativity.

However, it is facile to think that artistic creativity is separate from emotional creativity since, clearly, artistic expression and the artistic act are infused with the artist's emotional life – i.e., with his or her inner and outer life, with his/her capacity to tolerate the tension between 'reality' and 'illusion'. It would seem, rather, that in music therapy the issue is not so much to distinguish between 'art' and 'emotion', but rather to distinguish between 'art-and-emotion' that is generated *within* a relationship, and that which is generated outside a relationship. It is the relationship – the therapeutic relationship – that emphasises the primary creativity in music therapy, since the improvisation becomes the 'playground'. This playground provides a space within which the therapist and client can 'play', can test boundaries between the 'self' and the 'world', conveyed and portrayed here through and by the music. The nature of this jointly created dynamic form presents the client's capacity for autonomy, authenticity and playing. And by working (and playing) with this dynamic form, trying it out in different ways, breaking it up, regrouping it, stretching, shrinking and inverting it, the therapist and client together explore different ways of 'being in the world'.

One way of crystallising why we can be so sure that 'playing' music is the same as 'playing life', so to speak, is to interface musical and emotional creativity through the concept of dynamic form, discussed earlier. Dynamic form, as we saw, is embodied in clinical improvisation, where the common fabric between music and our feeling life is synthesised. The creation of sound form for emotional intent is neither a wholly musical nor a wholly emotional event. Rather the quality of the form is a consequence of its psychological function: to communicate, to explore, to express and receive all of these from and with another.

Within the space of clinical improvisation, the emotional and the musical are the same phenomenon, although a listener untrained to 'read' the emotional form may well hear the improvisation as a 'purely musical' event. In other words, although dynamic form is a synthesis of the musical and personal, it can be viewed (or listened to) from either the musical or the emotional side of the interface. Here we can think in terms of artistic creativity as being both similar to, and different from, emotional creativity. We can think in terms of each of these overlapping the other while at the same time extending beyond the other. In terms of clinical improvisation in music therapy, it might be helpful to think in terms of a paradox: the tension between their overlap and their separateness (Figure 11.1).

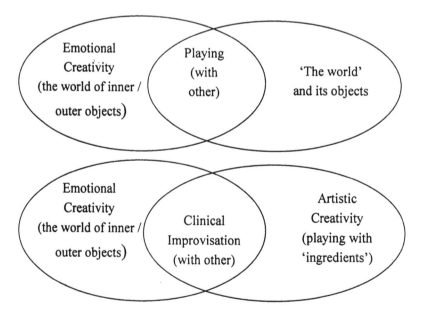

Figure 11.1 The parallels between 'playing' and clinical improvisation

Musing about Art

I want now to look at the interface between life and art from 'the other side', so to speak, and enter the domain of artistic creativity. Here, too, we see that music and the personal life are not as separate as they might seem, although the musical and the personal is a solitary, rather than an inter-personal, event. In reflecting on a musical composition, can we really listen to it as only a bunch of notes and rhythmic clusters woven together in an interesting or unusual way?

If we listen to what composers say about the process of artistic creativity, it seems that the need to create is not just a musical need, but has an emotional aspect that is at least as important, if not more so, as the musical one. This we can see as an extension of Winnicott's idea of primary creativity: the composer is creating a new experience of himself, using aspects of his personal, internal creation of the world and 'playing' with the external objects of musical sound to give the internal world external embodiment. Thus the act of composing music is far deeper than simply a need to 'play' with sounds, and in terms of 'playing' it is a solitary, rather than relational, activity.

The composers Aaron Copland (1952) and Igor Stravinsky (1974) use almost identical words to describe their experiences of composing music. Copland writes of the personal need to create: each new work brings with it an element of self-discovery, providing a unique formulation of his personal experiences. Stravinsky, though using less personal language than Copland, also speaks of the 'natural need' to compose. He describes the process of composition as a discovery, step by step, of the work he is creating as well as the discovery of himself. This process carries emotion for him, rather than bringing him purely intellectual gratification. Karlheinz Stockhausen (1974) speaks of the creative process as a powerful spiritual experience. Being in music transforms his whole existence – he moves towards becoming the sounds and becoming 'more timeless'. He himself enters the process, rather than creating a process that takes place outside of himself.

Stravinsky (1974) writes that he cannot simply compose music within a stylistic abyss, but needs external musical conventions to provide boundaries within which he can express himself. He speaks of needing a clearly defined, finite framework which can contain him – the thought of what he calls 'the abyss of total freedom' (p.64) in composition is 'terrifying'. It is clear that his terror is not just musical or artistic, but an emotional one: one that has to do with him as a human being. Composing music generates a process of self-expression which is profoundly personal – it draws from the depths of who he is – although it becomes transformed into a more conscious and formalised process (at this stage we might say that it is a craft). The process of composition culminates in a form that has cultivated aesthetic as well as emotional meaning, moving beyond the personal towards the universal. We might think of the two processes as being held in tension with one another: the composer's personal need and energy are tempered by external stylistic conventions of his period. The process of composition is meaningful for Stravinsky at a level which is more than just 'musical'.

Michael Tippett (1974) writes of being possessed by a creative drive from within, of imagining sounds and creating music from the inner world of his imagination. Like Stravinsky, he grapples to create order from chaos. He sees his function as a composer being, '...to continue an age-old tradition, fundamental to our civilisation... This tradition is to create images from the depths of the imagination and to give them form, whether visual, intellectual or musical. For it is only through images that the inner world communicates at all' (p.156).

It seems, then, that these 'purely musical' acts of musical composition are far from being purely musical. Rather they appear to be inseparable from the emotional process of the person creating the music: the act of composing offers a new synthesis of the self. However, here we are in the medium for 'artistic' creation – the creation of a work of art and, unlike clinical improvisation, this does not take place within the context of an interaction with another person (unless the composition is in the form of a group improvisation, as were many of Stockhausen's pieces); nor is the emotional form the end product of the creative activity. Rather, in composition, the striving is for an aesthetic of music: movement into 'new' musical territory, the trying out of different musical maps, so to speak, and this process is inseparable from the emotional forms of the composers that find realisation in the musical act of creation. As listeners, we then hear the musical form (to which we may, of course, assign emotional features). In the domain of the visual arts, we see that the same fusion of the personal and the artistic applies. Marion Milner (1957) suggests that painters conceptualise, non-verbally, through painting, '...the astounding experience of how it feels to be alive, the experience known from inside' (p.159). Kandinsky (1914), too, tells us that the goal of the artist is not merely 'mastery over form', but rather the act of painting, '...must be directed to the improvement and refinement of the human soul' (p.54).

Musing about Art and Emotion

It is worth clarifying that just because some music therapists speak about their sessions in 'purely musical' terms, this does not mean that the emotional aspect of the improvisation is sealed off, and that they are working exclusively through an 'artistic' medium, such as, e.g., composing music with clients. Rather it would seem that some therapists do not conceptualise the emotional aspect as detachable or separate from the musical act. It may be that they do not need to speak the language of 'emotion', and of emotional processes, but prefer to think and act therapeutically directly and only through music.

Thus when Gary Ansdell (1995) speaks of 'intrinsic interpretation', where, instead of interpreting through words the therapist responds within the pattern of the music itself – and this leads to the client (and therapist) finding something new within that shared musical experience – this does not mean that the feeling life is not engaged. It may mean that the interactive and inter-personal concepts remain musical, and the therapeutic integrity of the clinical improvisation is maintained, although some would question its depth. The absence of using psychodynamic language, and the use instead of musical language, does not always mean that the therapist and client are only tuning into music-as-music. However, in some instances, it may mean just this. When, in a case study presentation, the therapist speaks in terms of musical structure, musical style, idiom and form, then the listeners may well wonder whether the therapist and client are just 'playing music'. In psychodynamic terms, we could describe this 'purely musical' portrayal as a defence against the client and the therapist's feeling life by embracing and extending the improvisation only as an aesthetic, musical phenomenon. At the same time, just because the therapist and client 'do not speak' in sessions and engage purely through music, does not mean that the event is a purely musical one, devoid of personal relationship and personal meaning.

I had an experience of working only through music with a young man, 'Keith', who was a highly skilled pianist. The level and quality of our improvisatory skills totally seduced the musician in me. For the first two or three sessions I was filled with excitement and delight at our music-making. It took a while for me to realise that we were not 'doing' music therapy, but rather we were playing music. In my clinical supervision I developed a strong intuition that Keith's 'musical competence', and his seductive music, were a successful way of keeping me at bay, so to speak: they prevented a more intimate, intersubjective relationship from developing. I had simply no sense or feeling about how Keith felt while we played or, for that matter, before or after our playing. In the counter-transference I developed feelings of being marginalised, ineffectual, of not being needed by him. In this instance my attempts at sharing these insights verbally with Keith were unsuccessful. He simply did not hear. I was left – alone – to try and reach him and develop a more mutual relationship directly through the music. Not very successfully. In terms of our discussion, we might say that Keith was choosing to remain within the field of 'artistic' creativity, and sealing this from being influenced by 'emotional creativity' – hence my increasing discomfort and suspicion. In thinking about this from a psychodynamic perspective, his wonderful music was autonomous: he kept it to himself, and although its quality was emotional, this emotion was not authentically about 'me and him'. In other words, it was not a relational autonomy, that could both acknowledge me while still retaining a sense of himself.

However, at the same time, we cannot suggest that there is no artistic component in music therapy: on the contrary, clinical improvisation techniques place a large emphasis on creating music with the client that is as aesthetically pleasing as possible – while not compromising its clinical import.

Gary Ansdell (1995) asks whether therapeutic art is real 'art' – and whether the normal aesthetic standards apply to, say, clinical improvisation. If normal aesthetic standards do not apply, he then asks, has beauty anything to do with therapy? Can clinical improvisation be seen as an aesthetic object in its own right? Do we agree with Ansdell, when he says that any full understanding of it, as music therapy, demands also an aesthetic understanding? He points out that beauty is seldom mentioned as an element of therapy – perhaps because of an anxiety of appearing sentimental (and a leftover of the rather puritanical idea that beauty is 'bad' in contrast to the Ancient Greeks who saw beauty as 'good'). He speaks of moments of beauty, in his case studies, as being moments of transformation: moments that happened in 'real' music and that were Art (with a capital A).

Caroline Kenny's idea (cited in Aigen 1995) of a clinical aesthetic alerts us to the notion of beauty not only being the domain of the arts, but also as pertaining to the human person as a balanced, integrated, harmonious, engaging being. This needs to be extended towards beauty being generated between persons. The fluid and highly intimate engagement between therapist and patient may be seen as an event with a particular aesthetic quality, so that we can extend the idea of using art as a therapeutic medium to seeing the therapeutic process itself as an art form – a clinical art form. Both Aigen (1995) and Rose (1992) draw extensively from John Dewey's (1934) notion of the aesthetic as having to do as much with 'life' as with 'art'. It seems, though, that a distinctive feature of the aesthetic in clinical improvisation is not only about balance, integration and engagement. It is also about these as inter-personal qualities. In other words, the 'beauty' here is in the relationship.

I recall singing a Negro Spiritual with an African child from a severely disadvantaged background in a session. This child suddenly began to sing with a new passion – a profoundly moving moment of renewal, of conversion, of transformation – which was filled with beauty in a relational sense. It was not just that the song and his singing were beautiful; it was as if the child led me, showed me that this was where we could move towards, together. This moment shifted our relating to a new dimension, and here the beauty was an inter-personal beauty. The child's passion and intensity were shared and created in the space between us: although he led the way, I was part of the event. It was not autonomous, as in the case of Keith.

In group work, too, we can think of beauty in the way that a group of fragmented, dispersed children suddenly move and breathe together, during a movement-and-sound activity in group music therapy (Pavlicevic 1994). I agree with Ansdell that to think of beauty in clinical terms is not to sentimentalise or to diminish the therapeutic value of music therapy – but at the same time, beauty in a therapeutic sense may include dissonance, tension and fragmentation. Here it is the new authenticity, the extension towards a broader landscape, that is 'beautiful', potentially leading towards a new balance, integration and 'order'.

Taking Leave of Winnicott

Winnicott's reality, explored in this chapter, seems especially appropriate to music therapists, because of his interest in, and exploration of, the nature of creativity in human life. The next chapter leaves Winnicott aside and moves towards specific concepts drawn from psychodynamic theory. Before leaving Winnicott, though, it is worth remembering that although his language and concepts are enormously appealing to music therapists, and indeed to arts therapists in general, our indebtedness must be a clear one; one that does not simply 'borrow' or 'dip into' his theory, but that manages to reciprocate, contributing meaning to how we use his ideas as music therapists.

CHAPTER 12

Psychodynamic Meaning
in Music Therapy

Telling the truth and not telling it, and how much, is a lesser problem than the one of shifting perspectives, for you see your life differently at different stages, like climbing a mountain while the landscape changes with every turn of the path... Besides the landscape itself is a tricky thing. As you start to write at once the question begins to insist: Why do you remember this and not that? Why do you remember in every detail a whole week, month, more of a long ago year, but then complete dark, a blank? How do you know that what you remember is more important than what you don't?

(Doris Lessing, Under My Skin)

Doris Lessing reminds us that it is not only at the level of 'what something means' that we continue to evolve, uncover and shift meaning. It seems that even the fact itself, what we make of it, what we recall clearly, what we forget, and even where we are standing, influences its 'truth'.

In this chapter, psychodynamic concepts explore the diversity and shifts in meaning in relation to music therapy practice. Only some psychodynamic concepts are discussed, since this varied and rich field cannot begin to be addressed in these pages. These concepts are presented and discussed in order to clarify how a fact – an event – may come to have meaning that may be at once personal, interpersonal, elusive, exclusive, private and deeply hidden.

Interpretation

Interpretation in psychodynamic terms is usually understood as the therapist offering or suggesting to the client an understanding or insight that may clarify, for both therapist and client, an undeveloped or unexpressed meaning about an aspect of their work together. The therapist usually offers an interpretation after a private synthesis has begun to take place within the therapist, rather than only on the basis of a spontaneous feeling in response to the patient. In this sense, interpretation cannot be examined separately from counter-transference, which I shall explore later.

The timing, content and appropriateness of the interpretation are usually considered to be at least as important as the content of the interpretation itself. An inaccurate or badly timed interpretation by the therapist may result in the client withdrawing in some way from the relationship. For example, the client may take the inappropriate interpretation on board and go off at a tangent; the client may disagree directly with the therapist, may withdraw into impenetrable silence (in contrast to a softer, searching silence), and so on. In contrast, an interpretation that is apposite and congruent can uncover valuable connections between hitherto unrecognisable aspects about the client, or the client-and-therapist. Interpretation can be somewhat mystified by psychotherapists, many of whom set great store on its significance. Perhaps we can think of interpretation more in terms of a mutual exploration by therapist and client, than as something arrived at, and offered by, the therapist to the client.

Although in verbal psychotherapy, interpretation is usually verbal, it draws from both the verbal and non-verbal aspects of the therapist and client's work together.

Here I want to enquire into whether, in music therapy practice, interpretation features at all. Does interpretation need to be verbal – indeed, *ought* it to be verbal? Can we comfortably remain in the music, interpreting through the music, bypassing words altogether? It would be altogether too facile to think that since music is the primary medium of therapeutic encounter for many music therapists, interpretations need to occur exclusively through the music. Music and words are different modes of thinking and expressing, but can interpretations arising out of the musical act 'cross the line' into the verbal domain? Before exploring these issues, I want to reflect on various aspects of how we listen in music therapy, since I believe that this cannot be separated from how (and if) we interpret.

How we listen

The complexity of listening in creative music therapy has been touched on by Gary Ansdell (1995), who suggests that the therapist listens both to the music being improvised with the client and to the person (the other) in the music. We might say, rather, that the person *is* the music rather than the person being *in* the music. We have seen that clinical improvisation reveals dynamic forms of feeling: clinical improvisation reveals the essence of how the person is in the world, although the relationship is created by both players. The music is not about the person, it *is* the person. Perhaps, in terms of listening, the tension lies between the joint dynamic form of the musical relationship and the individuals that are part of that relationship: the relationship – the quality of the relationship – that reveals the individual within it. The person, we might say, does not exist outside the relationship. In order to gain a sense of the client through dynamic form, the therapist needs to be able to distinguish which aspects of the improvisation are hers and which are not. (But what does the client listen to? And how? As therapists we have the benefit of a training that enables us to read the joint improvisation for what it may reveal. The client has no such training, and may well hear a blur of sounds, 'noise' that is distressing, a 'nice wee tune', and so on.)

I suggest that we all listen differently at different times. During the act of playing, our listening is coloured by the immediate movement and physicality of the act, which feeds the acts of playing as it unfolds. We saw earlier that the act of listening is a perceptual/cognitive, as well as an emotional, act. There is a different quality to listening as the event draws to a close: here we listen to its 'echo', to the physical/musical/emotional pulses of both therapist and client settling. The music has just ended, the therapist and the client have accumulated impressions, musical images, sensations that may be on the threshold, barely formed, due to the movement only just coming to a close. Here the listening is still 'hot' – suffused with the immediacy of the jointly created music's colour and momentum, and whatever feelings the players have, will be coloured by this 'heat'.

We also listen to the session 'in our mind', so to speak, after the session has ended, music about 'how the session went'. In addition, many music therapists listen to a tape recording after the session. Here the quality of attention can be described as cooler, more objective in the sense of the therapist-listener being removed from the event, while being fed by its recalled kinetic and emotional imprint, and by other, non-musical impressions. We revisit feelings and intuitions that arose during the actual session, and are alert to new ones that arise during this 'second listening'.

The therapist can be said to synthesise all of these listening experiences when forming interpretations, but more than this, the therapist also listens to herself thinking emotionally and verbally. This listening contributes to the interpretation. Interpretation offered from this wide-ranging 'summit' draws from the entire panorama of listening, as well as from the 'different degrees of magnification' which Sandra Brown (1992) has explicated so succinctly. Brown describes the constant movements to and from the overview of therapy: these include termly summaries and reports, overviews of individual sessions, the indexing of the events in the sessions, and finally the minute musical details which music therapists hone in on, due to their clinical significance.

Interpretation: verbal and/or musical?

If we now turn our attention to interpretation in music therapy, we can think of interpreting directly through the music, and here Odell's (1989) assertion makes sense: that the therapist's anticipating and/or responding to the client through the music *in a certain way* is a form of interpretation. This is because the therapist's musical response or anticipation is based on listening (in all its dimensions) and acting upon clinical hunches as to 'what might be going on' between herself and the client. The therapist's clinical anticipation, revealed through the music, needs to be distinguished from a 'purely musical' anticipation. This means that the therapist's musical response and anticipation is not just about moving the music towards a more 'musical' improvisation. Rather it is a form of clinical sensing[1] embodied through music. The issue here is whether this interpretation arises from non-musical clinical concepts, or whether it is a music/feeling impulse that is coloured by clinical sensing.

But what if the interpretation is a verbal one? What if the therapist is drawn towards speaking with the client during a session? Here, the relating between therapist and client extends into another mode. While, in my experience, verbal interpretation can significantly shift the music improvisation towards a freer and more profound relating, as will be shown in a later example, it can also prevent the therapist and client from realising the full potential of the *musical*–therapeutic relationship.

There are obvious instances where talking is ineffectual and inappropriate, for example when working in the area of people suffering from delusions and hallucinations. Here, in my experience, words confuse the issue for the therapist and, I propose, for the client (Pavlicevic 1987). In work with clients who are non-verbal or pre-verbal, Ansdell's idea of 'intrinsic' interpretation, grounded in the concrete musical experience of 'doing', is a useful one, although I am not certain that the musical pattern can really be seen as being 'contentless' in the sense of being only itself. In instances such as these, what about the therapist's feelings? How do these feelings relate to the 'contentless' music? Therapists who work with profoundly handicapped people may feel exhausted, frustrated, despairing and even bored at times (Pavlicevic

---

1   The Oxford English Dictionary defines sensing as, 'the ability to perceive or feel or to be conscious of the presence or properties of things' (p.1103 OED 1990).

1995). Where do these feelings enter the equation of music being 'simply itself' in music therapy? Also, in working with profoundly handicapped people who may 'do' very little in sessions, can the music, created mostly by the therapist, be 'removed' from her feelings and be convincingly seen as 'contentless'?

There is another aspect to do with working with this client group. If the therapist chooses to read the musical event psychodynamically, and make interpretations, does she interpret to herself? How can this interpretation be shared with the client? Where the therapist interprets with her supervisor, this may well result in a shift in the music-making in the client's presence. Here we might think in terms of a 'musical' interpretation, as described by Odell (1989). Despite the interpretation being a solitary act that cannot be shared verbally with the client, the therapist acts musically upon her 'private' interpretation and searches for resonance from the patient. Where the client is severely handicapped, the client's responsive cues may be extremely subtle, as in slight changes in body movements or breathing. This resonance may be experienced by the therapist herself, in a shift of feelings about and towards the client during the session.

Bringing to consciousness

There is another aspect to interpretation that needs some reflection: this is the issue of 'bringing to consciousness'. If client and therapist remain only in the musical act, and the therapist interprets only through music, can the musical act itself come to have a full conscious meaning for the client? Is there a musical 'consciousness' that somehow infuses into 'verbal' consciousness? Do we say that the meaning of the act only becomes fully conscious when it is verbalised? Sometimes, in clinical improvisations, clients 'know' that 'something' has happened. They cannot verbalise it, their knowing is musically based, in the sense that its context is the act of playing. Does this kind of 'knowing' signify a shift from the unconscious to conscious life – or do we need words in order to explicate? (And is it 'mechanistic' to think of conscious and unconscious as adjacent entities, with various degrees of permeability?)

Art therapist David MacLaggan (1994) suggests that the link between the artistic image and its unconscious significance is often assumed. But how is this assumption made; how does it come about? And if we want to ensure that we do not assume this link, how do we find the language to 'fit' the phenomenon and avoid too many assumptions? How do we find a language that captures, at once, the image, as well as its more distant, undefinable qualities? In music therapy, this language needs to do justice to the interactive complexities, to the musical inter-dynamic, and to the unconscious meaning of any feature of these aspects of the therapeutic event, as well as to the whole event. As such, interpretation, whether through words or music, is exploratory. It is a creative act in itself. It is also a mutual act in that both patient and therapist, together, find meaning.

Finally we need to consider whether, in fact, interpretation is always necessary. Patrick Casement's (1995) encouragement to sustain a harmonious binocular vision, where we both know and do not know, is salutary. We need to guard against making interpretations purely because of our theoretical leanings, or because we have read somewhere that interpretation is central to the therapist–client relationship. We need to guard against the pressure of interpreting as a way of reassuring ourselves that we 'know what is going on'.

Transference

At its most general, transference has to do with feelings that the patient transfers on to the therapist, and some music therapists speak of a transference relationship between client and instrument in music therapy (Towse 1991). These feelings are usually understood to be echoes of the patient's past, often having to do with 'unfinished business'. For example, there may exist in the patient unresolved feelings about, say, his mother. The therapist represents to the patient a 'figure of authority' (in the broadest sense), and, as such, evokes in him a certain way of being towards the therapist. For example, the patient may feel judged and criticised by the therapist, or may feel that the therapist is bored with him. This way of being and of feeling towards the therapist may have little to do with the actual personality of the therapist (the therapist may be open and accepting of the patient and very interested in him), but rather the patient's feelings have to do with his emotional perception of the therapist as a figure of authority. This may resonate with the patient's own mother who was indeed critical and judgmental.

Transference is usually considered to be part of any psychotherapeutic encounter. The emergence and existence of feelings felt by the patient towards the therapist are explored by therapist and patient where possible, and this enables the patient to access and address forgotten events and feelings. These forgotten feelings may stem from the patient's pre-verbal life (what Freudians call the pre-Oedipal level), or they may be from later events that have been repressed, denied and tucked away in the patient's unconscious.

Some psychoanalysts distinguish between the quality of remembering, and of repressing of events that occurred in the patient's pre-verbal life and those that occurred after the acquisition of language. Joyce McDougall writes:

> With regard to traumatic events stemming from even earlier periods, before the acquisition of *verbal* communication, the detection of their existence becomes considerably more complicated – to the point that we may only become aware of the traumatic dimension through the unconscious pressure it exerts on the analysand's way of being and speaking, and thus may eventually only be accessible if captured through our *countertransference reactions* (1993, p.96).

And yet it seems that events that occurred after the acquisition of language and the capacity for verbal thought are by no means more straightforward to unravel. Joyce McDougall clarifies that verbally shaped memories can severely limit the significance of the remembered experience: 'Such events when recounted in the course of the analysis often present themselves as unshakeable facts, rather than as thoughts and free associations that can be explored psychically, and as such they serve the function of resistance to the unfolding of the analytic process' (McDougall 1993, p.96).

Patrick Casement (1985) talks of a transference as having to do with *similarity* between past and present experiences: he suggests that it is the misperception by the patient of similarity as sameness that triggers the phenomenon of transference in the patient. In other words, something in the present has a similarity to something in the past, but the patient misperceives the similarity as being the same as the past. As a result, the patient transfers from the past, previous experiences and feelings, and relives them as if they were in the present. Casement stresses the importance of allowing space and time for the patient to discover his feelings, and, through them, to discover the distinguishing differences between the past, the present, and the past that spills into the present.

Counter-transference

Counter-transference is complicated. Broadly speaking, counter-transference describes the emotions that the therapist develops towards the client in response to the client in sessions. The sources of these feelings are wide-ranging and rather complex, and it is because of these complexities that therapists and analysts need to undergo their own psychotherapy/analysis. The therapist needs to be able to discern what aspects of her feelings of counter-transference are to do with her own unresolved issues, what aspects have to do with what Jungian analyst, Adolf Guggenbuhl-Craig (1971) describes as the 'newly accessed' shadow aspects of the therapist as a result of working with the client. Aspects of counter-transference may also have to do with feelings that have been put there, into the therapist, by the client.

Unacknowledged counter-transference may cause the therapist to listen to the patient 'narrowly', from within the confines of a theoretical orientation; it may result in the therapist pre-empting the patient, by reaching a 'conclusion' as a result of a false sense of recognition in the patient's communication. The therapist may have a 'transferential' attitude to the patient's lateness (as anger or resistance), to silence in the session (as withholding or resisting) or around expressing anger. All of these may leave the therapist deaf to unexpected revelations.

Counter-transference is a valuable clinical tool which the psychotherapist is trained to recognise as revealing valuable information about the patient. In this sense the therapist's response to the patient may be informed by the counter-transference. Through reflecting on feelings of counter-transference, the therapist may gain critical insights into 'what is going on' in the session, and in the patient's life. However, because of the complexity of transference and counter-transference, therapists typically search for support in their work, in the form of supervision. Here they can be supported in their search to be as receptive and responsive to the patients as they are able.

Transference, Counter-transference and Music Therapy

Diaz de Chumaceiro (1992) acknowledges that while the ubiquitousness of transference and counter-transference, as well as the diversity of understandings, may seem overwhelming to music therapists who are not psychoanalytically oriented, she cautions strongly against ignoring it, on that basis.

I now want to draw from some clinical music therapy work in an attempt to gain clarity on transference and counter-transference in this context.

In music therapy work with a gifted musician called 'Jayne', I experienced strong feelings of 'my hands being tied': I felt clinically unable to develop or extend what and how we played. Every avenue that I attempted to explore was adeptly blocked by Jayne, through the music. I felt powerless. Powerless both musically and personally. As a result of this I began to feel frustrated and exasperated with Jayne. These strong feelings were examined in my supervision: where did they come from and what did they mean? I needed to tease out feelings that stemmed directly from the music, that had to do with me, the musician, feeling frustrated and constrained, and personal feelings of frustration. All of these feelings belonged to the clinical situation, but not all belonged to the clinical relationship between me and Jayne. Was there something about her person that triggered something in me? Was this a trigger from my past? Something about feeling powerless? About feeling controlled, and not coping with feeling controlled? This did not feel quite right when I explored it in my supervision, so I then explored from a different position: were my clinical responses appropriate for her? Was my music really meeting her in the way that she needed to be met? I was not sure that it was, and this prompted further exploration.

My supervisor and I then explored what this was telling me about her, about us. As we spoke and explored, I began to feel more and more as though some of my feelings of powerlessness and the resulting frustration had to do with part of who and how I am as a human being, and part had to do with the clinical context. It seemed increasingly that I was experiencing feelings that belonged to the client: her *own* feelings of powerlessness and being out of control were being channelled through me – in psychodynamic terms we would say that these were feelings that she had projected *into* me.[2] Feelings that were unconscious and unbearable, and that she passed into me so that I could experience them for her, try them out, so to speak.

As a result of insights gained with the support of my supervisor, Jayne and I were able to verbalise the feelings between us: I said that I felt powerless and that my hands were tied. She then spoke of feeling that I, as therapist, had 'the power', and that I was the one who 'directed'. She spoke of feeling stuck and of wanting to be together in a way that was mutual, but of feeling that she was unable to do so. As soon as she said this, something between us shifted: it was as though a new dynamic had been set in motion by verbally developing what had been going on musically. I then remembered aloud that at the end of a previous session, I had suggested that we do a 'quick' piano duet to finish off. I had asked whether she would like me to give her an ostinato (which is not at all my *modus operandi*). She had been enthusiastic, and there had followed some two minutes of gloriously playful, animated playing from both of us. It had been great fun. I reminded her of this and she agreed that it had been a highlight of our work together so far. I then wondered aloud whether this was because of the predetermined musical structure, which made her feel that it was not I, the therapist, in control of

---

2   There is a distinction between projecting feelings *on to* a person and projecting them *into* someone. Feelings that are unconscious and unbearable are often projected on to persons whom we do not know well and who fulfil certain criteria, such as belonging to an ethnic minority, a different social class, a different age group. They are our scapegoats who can carry our unbearable feelings for us. However, we may project unconscious unbearable feelings *into* someone with whom we are on intimate terms: this enables them to carry the feelings for us, and almost to 'try them out' for us. We can then be assured that these feelings are 'bearable' by another person, and as therapist we can pass back the projected feelings to the client.

the music, but rather that the pre-negotiated structure determined it. She concurred enthusiastically, and I then asked whether she wanted us, together, to set a structure on to our music improvisations, as we had done with the previous duet. She felt that this would help. With hindsight, I now see that I was being rather literal.

In the event, we did not, of course, need to negotiate or predetermine a musical structure. Our talking through what had been going on in the music enabled the energy between us to shift, and this was reflected in subsequent musical improvisations. A feeling of companionship and mutuality was able to be expressed between us, and the remainder of our work together was much more 'honest', in the sense that when either of us experienced feeling stuck with one another, or when either of us felt that something significant had happened, we were able, increasingly, to share it. In terms of our struggling together to find a mode of working that was comfortable to us both, rather than my continuing to keep my frustrations to myself, Irvin Yalom's (1989) words are affirming: 'Though there is something reassuring about an omniscient therapist who is always in control of every situation, there can be something powerfully engaging about a fumbling therapist, a therapist willing to flounder with the patient until they, together, stumble upon an enabling discovery' (p.36).

In terms of transference and counter-transference, we can understand the following from this example. The client had certain feelings about the therapist. These feelings (of powerlessness[3]) belonged *both* to the client and to the therapist, in that the therapist may well have been over-directive and 'powerful'. This made the client feel powerless, which may have amplified her experience of the therapist as a figure of authority.

Let us use Patrick Casement's explanation, discussed earlier, to try and unravel this a little. Casement suggests that one way of understanding transference is to consider the client as misperceiving similarity with sameness. Thus the experience by the client of the therapist as a figure of authority was *similar to* other figures of authority in the client's life. The client, however, may have experienced the therapist's authority as *being the same as* the authority of, let us say, her father/mother/teachers. It was this experiencing of the therapist as being the same as, rather than being similar to, that resulted in the client's experiencing the therapist *not* as a person 'only in the present', but as someone with feelings that belonged to the client's past. These feelings

---

3   The feelings were more complex than those on the spectrum of power versus
    powerlessness, but I choose to limit this discussion to these.

of powerlessness were unbearable to the client and were, at this point, unconscious. Because of the existing therapeutic relationship, the client projected these feelings into the therapist. The therapist experienced feelings of being stuck and of being powerless, although her initial cues were musical ones. At this point, we can say that the therapist experienced feelings of counter-transference – these feelings, in part, gave rise to the therapist's feelings of frustration.

Why do we say this and how can we be sure? Through clinical supervision, the therapist was able to see that some of these feelings did not entirely belong to her. She felt uncomfortable and frustrated, but the quality of those feelings did not quite 'fit' with how she usually experiences herself as a person. By carefully and thoroughly exploring the possibilities, the therapist was able to tease out those aspects of the feelings which belonged to her. These needed to be put to one side, so to speak, so as not to let them interfere with what was going on between her and the client at the time. By fully acknowledging, and putting them aside, the therapist was able to be fully 'there for' the client. The therapist then acted verbally on the counter-transference by speaking to the client about feeling stuck and wondering how the client was feeling and did any of these feelings resonate with her? It is important to remember, here, that the therapist might have conveyed her insights within the improvisation – that is, without speaking. I did not know how to do this.

We can draw encouragement from the writings of those who support us in our state of 'unknowing'. This permits us to be vulnerable and unknowing with our clients (rather than maintaining a confident persona of 'knowing' with clients, and then revealing our uncertainties in supervision, 'behind their backs', so to speak). Patrick Casement (1985) is volubly enthusiastic about maintaining what he calls an openness to the unknown, or a state of 'harmonious mix-up'. He suggests that there exists a creative tension between knowing and not knowing that the therapist needs to be able to tolerate, along with feelings of ignorance, uselessness and incompetence. Similarly, Harry Guntrip (1971) urges us to be fully ourselves with our clients, rather than just a professional. He writes: '...the analyst must be a whole real human being with the patient and not just a professional interpreter of the patient's psychic life. Only then can the patient find himself and become a person in his own right' (p.66).

Music, Words, Consciousness

The process just described crossed into verbal dialogue with the client. But what about acting purely musically? It seems critical to understand that aspects of these phenomena may indeed be acted upon only through the music, and here my sense is that the musical act needs to be informed, and coloured, by the searching described above. I want to draw from another example to illustrate this.

A woman called 'Rose' always churned out one pretty, schmaltzy tune after the other in our sessions. My intuition was that this music was 'inauthentic' – we could say that the tunes were a defence against her more 'real' music, of which I had only an intuitive inkling, but a strong one. Informed by my increasing feelings of boredom with the falseness of this music, my musical responses to her began to change: I ceased 'going along with' the pretty tunes that she churned out. I began, instead, to colour her tunes with quite different harmonic textures: at first very subtly introducing dissonant intervals (e.g. major 7th, augmented 4th), introducing fairly bland cross-rhythms (e.g., 6/8 to her 3/4, or 2/4 to her 6/8) that slanted the tunes somewhat differently, while all the time being alert to how this felt to me and to how she responded musically. I had a sense of personal relief at no longer feeling the need to collude with the false prettiness. Eventually our joint music-making became more potent, more forceful. Gradually an astonishing eruption of passion and vitality took over our music-making. This, I felt, was nearer the mark – our mark. It was here that both of us were more fully and authentically ourselves with one another.

What interested me about this work was that the client remained, to some extent, unwilling to talk in the sessions. Our more momentous sessions, when the music was 'spectacular', in the sense of authentic energy and flexible passion, often brought forth a quiet, casual 'thank you, see you next week' at the end of the session, despite my obvious excitement. (I would often do a small dance to express my excitement once she had left the music room, as I could barely contain the sheer physicality of our music.) Clearly, though, she did not seem to need, or want to own, her vitality and passion verbally.

Does this mean, however, that she could not own her vitality and passion *consciously?* That even though the shift was significant, the fact that it happened only in the music meant that it remained unconscious? Do we tend to confuse musical meaning with unconscious meaning? Can consciousness be a purely musical phenomenon? Do we need to remove ourselves from the experience, talk about it, think about it, to render it more forceful? Do we agree with Reik (cited earlier by Odell 1989), who says that something not expressed verbally risks 'disappearing'?

My sense is that this is too simple an explanation. At the end of the work, Rose said that she was aware of 'things happening', but she did not know what these were or what they meant. I knew that 'things had happened', through the potent change in our music-making, but clearly, this knowledge was to remain in the realm of the unstated – for us both. However, I would not for a moment entertain that leaving the meaning verbalised and inexplicit means that it did not exist – and that her own shifts were not powerful. At the same time, though, I am not certain that, had we talked, she would have 'owned' these shifts more fully. It felt right not to speak – and certainly the potency of the improvisation lingered into the silences after playing, so that to then 'speak' could have been a 'defence against' allowing this (silent) potency to breathe. By talking, we might have wrapped the music up, put it aside, and 'talked'. We shall never know – and much of this remains paradoxical and, to some extent, inconclusive.

David John (1995) suggests that the process of what he calls 'free improvisation' on instruments is not unlike free association in psychoanalysis. The patient is encouraged to 'release a stream of sounds' (p.160), which have varying degrees of organisation and carry varying degrees of affect. This process, John suggests, enables the patient to find his 'pre-verbal' voice, and to communicate and discharge it into the therapist-as-container. In this way primitive feelings can become 'mastered' and more under conscious control. Is he then suggesting that the act of playing, of 'communicating and discharging', only goes as far as free-associating, without moving to the next step, which is 'bringing to consciousness'? Does the act remain, at a pre-verbal, rather than a non-verbal level? Does the 'free' improvisation enable a synthesis? Does the therapist interpret musically, verbally, or both?

Perhaps the distinctive feature of clinical improvisation is that it is a *joint* musical occurrence between two people that reveals particular forms of relating and of 'being with' and these may include 'discharging'. Powerful movements are effected through the musical interplay, during which the therapist holds, contains, nurtures and supports, and is 'being with' the patient. As such, the event itself is complete, and to *talk* about it with the patient may well detract and distract from the experience. For example, after an especially dark, murky and cloying improvisation with a depressed patient in an adult psychiatric hospital, I asked her how she found the music we had just played: her response was that it had been most relaxing, a 'jolly wee tune'. Although there was nothing interpretive about our verbal exchange, I have often wondered whether, by inviting her to talk about it, I removed her from the direct feeling experience of what we had just done together. At the same time, though, her comment gave me a valuable insight into how she managed her feelings.

Perhaps it is when there is an element of discomfort, of incompleteness, of incongruence or of puzzlement about what is going on, that the therapist and/or the patient will be moved to attempt words in sessions – as I did, in the earlier example with 'Jayne'. Perhaps, though, it is also when therapist and client want, and need, to extend the relationship into verbal mode.

What Kind of Consciousness?

To return to the question of consciousness, let us briefly revisit our earlier discussion on words and music (Figure 12.1). We have seen that the feelings between therapist and client are not only musical feelings (e.g. earlier we looked at feelings of frustration, boredom and powerlessness). These feelings may be *generated* by the musical act and may have a separate, non-musical life, which continues after the musical event has ended.

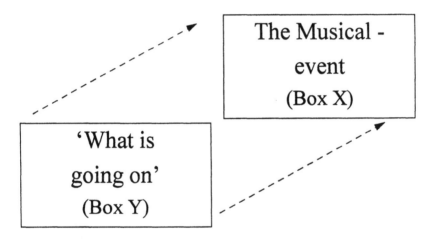

Figure 12.1 The relationship between what we do in music and how we understand it.

If we ignore Box Y, and simply look at what is going on in musical terms – in other words, we remain in box X – we can see that, in the work with the previous client, Jayne, the therapist tried certain musical avenues and the client blocked them. By exploring the musical minutiae we find that, for example, it was when the therapist played such-and-such a note that this seemed to trigger off Jayne negatively. We might then suggest different musical avenues, and try them out to see which might trigger the patient in a way that enhances the musical relationship and spectrum of intensity. While there is no reason why this approach would not work – and, indeed, this is the narrow and rather fundamentalist view of Nordoff–Robbins music therapy – I am certain that music therapists would agree that this is a limiting and limited way of working. And in any case, whether the therapist acknowledges it or not, the client's transference still affects the therapist's acts and skews them in a certain way. Transference and counter-transference do not only exist because the therapist understands, acknowledges and explores these processes. In other words, Box Y is part of Box X.

It would seem that, in thinking about the work in only a musical way, the whole person is not taken into account. Rather, the person is being seen only through the lens of their musical act. With Rose, even though we remained in the music, my work was informed by extra-musical nuances, understandings and reflections.

While the 'purely musical' picture (Box X) may, indeed, provide essential insights into the client's life, and while working only through this lens may indeed be highly effective, it can also be a way of the therapist not taking her own feelings into account. The therapist can 'absent' herself, her personal self, so to speak, and describe the work only in terms of who did what, when musically.

Let us return to how the client makes the therapist feel. Let us pretend that the therapist is bored by a client, dreads the weekly sessions, the work is going nowhere, the client does the same thing, week in week out. What does this scenario mean? How does this meaning inform the quality of the relationship – even when the relationship is understood to be a *musical* one? Can the therapist's feelings be non-existent, in the interests of 'pure' music therapy, that is, can we leave Box Y out of the picture? I think not. A scenario such as this is also, of course, unwittingly playing out both a transference and counter-transference: part of the therapist's unacknowledged counter-transference may be a discomfort with looking at the extra-musical 'feeling life' of either therapist or patient, which then results in a reluctance on theoretical grounds to explore this through words and, if appropriate, of sharing, verbally, explorations with the client.

However, as we saw in the work with Rose, the acknowledgement by the therapist of these feelings, and the exploration and eliciting of their meanings, need not result in verbalising. That which is acknowledged (Box Y)can be portrayed through music, not necessarily literally or directly – we might think more in terms of this 'colouring' the musical relationship. Thus the music therapist who does not want to consider the psychodynamic processes that are there in the music, irrespective of the therapist's awareness and 'belief', needs to consider the meaning of this reluctance.

In conclusion, music therapists need to be careful when and if supporting or dismissing the use of psychodynamic concepts. We need to ensure that we are not using 'working only in the music' as a shield behind which to conceal our 'selves', or that we are shielding poor musical-therapeutic work behind complex psychodynamic explanations. The grave risk is that we might offer the client only the 'musician-therapist', or the 'therapist-therapist', rather than the 'person-therapist who works in music'. The quality of the relationship will be lesser, for that.

CODA

CHAPTER 13

Why Do We Become Therapists?

If you can help others it is very good
Yet if you cannot do this,
At least do not harm them

(HH *The Dalai Lama, Taming the Tiger, 1989)*

Many music therapists go to great lengths, and spend a lot of energy, time and thought, in not just 'doing' music therapy, but also in thinking, talking and writing about it, this book being a case in point. Much writing about music therapy is based on our direct and personal experiences of clinical work with clients. We describe, and theorise about, clinical material from the sessions; we may contextualise our work within a broader treatment model and theoretical background; we may contextualise the work in the ethos of the school, clinic, hospital or day centre in which we work; we may focus on work with persons who suffer from a particular syndrome and find common threads, or on aspects of the therapist–client relationship. We write case studies, research reports or general theoretical musings that arise directly out of clinical experience (Bunt and Hoskyns 1987; Rogers 1995; Wheeler 1995).

In concluding this book, I want to explore why it is that, although music therapists continue to do the work and to search for meaning in the clinical work, we do not seem to spend much time exploring why we choose to become therapists in the first instance, and music therapists in particular. The question, it seems to me, is a large one.

Our motives for wanting to work in the 'helping professions' are, no doubt, complex and multi-layered. We may carry a wish to heal, to care and to accompany someone on their journey or share in an aspect of their life. We may be motivated by spiritual or religious beliefs, by a particular ideology

– or we may 'feel' that we want to 'be' music therapists. Many of us express the enormous richness, privilege and fulfilment in our roles: our work is vocational, drawing from our personal depths and resources, and affecting us accordingly: music therapy is both energising and draining. Somewhere along the way, however, we need to face the fact that the role of carer and healer, carries with it the potential for power and for self-delusion. This chapter attempts to explore the 'dark' side of being a therapist.

We might begin this exploration by asking ourselves the following: why do we choose to surround ourselves with those who are labelled as being 'ill', who are 'in need', who are 'handicapped' or 'disabled' in some way, who are 'disturbed' and who are 'mad'? By engaging with those who are classified as 'worse off' than we are, do we gain a sense of being 'better off', of being balanced, helpful, do-gooder? If this is so, why is it that we need to experience these positive sentiments about ourselves so explicitly, so unsubtly and in such polarity? Do we need to be able to have access to, to control an aspect in, the life of another who is 'weaker', 'less resilient', who is 'ill'?

The Wounded Healer

The Jungian analyst Adolf Guggenbuhl-Craig (1971), unfolds piercingly the shadow aspect of who and how we are as therapists, whether social workers, physicians, analysts, lawyers or priests. Many of us, he says, choose our profession out of a deep personal need. He reflects within the Jungian image of archetypes, which he describes as:

> '...an inborn potentiality of behaviour. Human beings react archetypally to someone or something when faced with a typical, constantly recurring situation. A mother or father reacts archetypally to a son or daughter, a man reacts archetypally to a woman, etc.... The basic situation of the archetype contains a polarity' (p.89).

James Hillman (1975) describes archetypes as metaphors rather than concrete images, and sees them as governing all perspectives of ourselves, the world, our behaviour and attitudes, and our unconscious. In this sense, we might think of archetypes as 'embryonic', taking shape when they connect with, and are activated by, an image or an event.

Guggenbuhl-Craig tells us that we contain both poles of an archetype rather than only one side or polarity, although we may only activate one aspect of the archetype. For example, we contain both poles of the parent–child, the healer–sick, the teacher–pupil archetypes, rather than simply containing the healer–archetype or patient–archetype. When we become ill, the healer–patient archetype is constellated or activated within us. Not only do we then need an external healer to help us get better, but we need to activate our own internal healer. This intra-psychic healer in the ill person is often known as the 'healing factor'. Someone who is gravely ill needs to have 'the will to live' if they are to survive and recover from their illness (Guggenbuhl-Craig p.90) – they need to activate their own, internal, healer.

However, our psyches often find it difficult to tolerate the tension in containing the two polarities (healer–patient) of the archetype, and one way of dealing with this tension is to repress one polarity of the archetype within ourselves. This means that the repressed polarity may continue to operate in our unconscious, for the most part leaving us alone, or we may project it on to the outer world. Thus someone who becomes ill, and who cannot tolerate both poles of the healer–patient archetype, can project his inner and repressed healer on to the doctor – which may result in the patient handing over his or her own healing factor, and relying on the doctor and nurses to do the 'curing'. Similarly, the healer who cannot tolerate both the healer–patient ends of that archetype, may either project his/her 'wounds' on to the patient, or they may repress the patient pole of the archetype. This can result in the healer gaining the impression that weakness and illness have only to do with the patient, and nothing to do with him or herself. The wounds belong to the patients. The healer then becomes 'only-doctor', healthy and strong, while the patients become 'only-patients', sick and weak. At the same time the healer is drawn, vocationally, to being the 'healer', in order to experience him or herself in tension (and in harmony) with the 'wounded'. The 'wounded' are positioned out there, well away from the healer, and they resonate with his or her own suppressed or projected woundedness. The 'only-healer' needs 'only-patients' to fulfil him or her.

In contrast is the healer who is aware of sickness as the counterpole of health, who has a constant awareness of his or her own degeneration of body and mind, and is truly the 'wounded healer'. This healer is the patient's brother/sister/friend/accompanist, rather than the patient's 'manager'. Although we all have within us the illness–health archetype, Guggenbuhl-Craig suggests that those of us who choose the healing professions have a special interest in, and are especially drawn towards, the illness–health, or healer–patient archetype: we want to – indeed, we need to – experience it directly. This need is what makes our work a vocational one, rather than purely job/career-oriented work.

Extending Ourselves

As part of our therapy training, we are taught to be sensitive and alert to the 'woundedness' of clients. We learn, for instance, about clinical conditions, abnormal development and about 'pathology'. Our practice focuses on the client – on 'the other'. We are there in order to heal the client. And yet our own needs are there: not only our needs in choosing to be therapists but also our ongoing needs within the therapeutic relationship. It seems that the less we pay attention to these needs, the less willing we are to embrace the 'shadow' side of our work, and the more likely we are to think of ourselves only as 'therapists' and turn patients into only 'patients'.

James Hillman (1975) exhorts us to exercise extreme caution to ensure that, as therapists, we are not using our clients as a vehicle or mirror to facing the darkness and woundedness within us. Doing this potentially takes care of, and absolves us from, undergoing our own journey into our inner darkness. He suggests that we need to own, and be aware of, the counter-transference that exists in us as therapists before the therapeutic encounter takes place. Because we are 'therapists' and the patient is a 'patient', we are oriented a certain way towards someone who is 'ill', thinking, for example, 'what is wrong?' and 'how can I help?'.

In thinking and reading around this topic, I began, once again, to question my own journey as a music therapist. Like many confident, altruistic young persons, I wanted to 'do good', and music therapy was the obvious path for a musician. The 'obstacles' – or the dark side of the work (which of course were the dark side of myself, although I did not know it at the time) – soon confronted me. When I began to work with profoundly and multiply handicapped people in Scotland, I had overwhelming feelings of nausea and exhaustion, and was frequently ill. I then met my first 'violent' patient – a 'crazy' young woman of mild mental handicap. I was paralysed with fear, certain that she would attack me at the earliest opportunity. Of course, at the time, I saw that all the 'violence' was in the patient: safely out there, somewhere, away from me. I felt safest, and the most enabling, with the mute, profoundly mentally disabled but physically 'normal' young men and women, who could satisfy my need to feel that I was the enabler – and who did not trigger my own darknesses. Their perceived 'benignness' resonated with my rather limited experience of myself as a benign, 'good' person. This was, however, a narrow resonance, and within two years I was bored with this work.

Then came a stint in an adult psychiatric hospital, where at first I was anxious about 'madness'. What did it mean, how did it sound, to be mad? Insidiously and steadily, while my initial apprehensions shifted towards excitement, fascination, and a caring and tenderness towards the wonderful people with whom I worked, I began to feel emotionally drained, physically ill and, at times, grey with fatigue. Clearly there was something in all that 'madness' that caused enormous inner stress, manifested somatically.

If we examine these events in terms of the shadow and the darkness alluded to earlier, we can attempt to see what was going on. As the 'healer', I was unable to tolerate my own inner wounds and needed to keep them tightly stitched. 'Mad' people could 'play out' my own madness for me, out there, and I could remain 'sane' – although I paid the price somatically. Until I began to work at reuniting the splits within myself – the splits of madness/sanity, formed/deformed, violence/peacefulness – I needed to remain 'in control': the therapist who could 'objectify' illness or handicap or violence as something 'out there'. I would listen out for it in the music, 'catch it', work with it and write compelling music therapy reports. I am certain that my work was extremely limited, despite bringing momentary satisfaction and a sense of achievement, at an 'ego' level.

It seems that working in the field of the conscious and the unconscious, makes us especially susceptible to our own unconscious. Guggenbuhl-Craig puts it as a psychological 'law': the more we strive for something bright, he says, the more its dark counterpart is activated. It is as though our psychic map has more territory on it precisely because our work is about bringing into consciousness our patients' unconscious states and processes. The more we develop our own conscious life, the more there is a corresponding unconscious. We need to be extra vigilant to our own vast darknesses.

Thus by accepting the woundedness within us, we become more human, more real as healers. Peter Hawkins and Robin Shohet (1989) put it thus:

> We have found that when we have been able to accept our own vulnerability and not defend against it, it has been a valuable experience both for us and our clients. The realisation that they could be healing us, as much as the other way round, has been very important both in their relationship with us and their growth. It is another reminder that we are servants of the process. (p.14)

It is interesting that it is now, many years later, that I am filled with doubts about my clinical work: I wonder, for instance, who is being the therapist and who is being the client; I recognise that I need music therapy – and, indeed, if I do not practise for any length of time, I miss it: the intensity, dynamism, directness: these are my needs, coupled with needing to be valued, to be seen as 'helping'.

Why Be Healthy?

In our 'reasonable' and medicalised world, there is a splendid distinction between illness and health, polarised from one another. In other words, am I healthy if I am ill?

In many parts of the world, there exist aspirations to what can be described as a 'grotesque' healthiness, which embraces the 'body beautiful', mindful logic and theraped psyches. Illness can be isolated; our 'symptoms' can be grouped and, more significantly, named. My illness has a name: I have cancer, 'flu', I suffer from schizophrenia, from a bipolar illness, a broken ankle, I am an abuse survivor, and so on. Once my symptoms are named, I can hand them over; to the professionals, the carers. They, who have named my symptoms and are experts, can cure me of it and make me healthy once again. There is simply no room for lunacy, for death, for suffering in our unpeculiar, homogeneous, sane world.

René Descartes is usually pinpointed as being responsible for the many splits in our culture. In terms of his influence on medicine, Ivan Illich (1976) writes:

> His description effectively turned the human body into clockworks and placed a new distance, not only between soul and body, but also between the patient's complaint and the physician's eye. Within this mechanised framework, pain turned into a red light and sickness into mechanical trouble. A taxonomy of diseases became possible. As minerals and plants could be classified, so diseases could be isolated and categorised by the doctor-taxonomist. (p.166)

Is this where we want to be as music therapists? Traditionally, many music therapists contextualise the work within the realm of 'pathology'. We work with the mentally or physically handicapped, with the mentally ill, with the terminally ill, with neurologically impaired people. We are employed in (special) schools, hospitals, clinics, day centres, community centres, and are acknowledged for our willingness to accommodate, and be part of, the medical model. We are beholden to the medical model for assuming that something is 'wrong'. We care, we support, we nurture, we guide, we treat, we 'improve the quality of a person's life', we 'alleviate symptoms'. And economic pressures and responsibilities confine us to ensuring that we can show 'improvement' and, with some luck, even remove 'pathology'. (Alternatively, we can sweep pathology aside altogether and speak of music therapy as providing 'peak experience', as part of growth, as offering experiences that transcend the baser aspects of life.)

Medicine and science acknowledge the value of music therapy, and may even be slightly puzzled by it: after all, music has been proven to affect the heart rate, the limbic system, mood states, and states of tension and relaxation in the body, so there must be something in it. Also, its musical/artistic basis arouses enthusiasm – as well as something approaching ambivalence – can art really have a place in the neon-lit world of medicine and science?

In the energetic conversations between James Hillman and Michael Ventura (Hillman and Ventura 1992), Hillman lambasts the 'mediocre' profession of psychotherapy for having encouraged a private 'hogging the psyche'. Why, he asks, do we tend to assume that the psyche is only within our skins? Why does psychotherapy grudgingly extend (Hillman uses the word 'condescend') to include the family and, perhaps here and there, the workplace, the 'organisation' – while the world 'out there' is left denuded of soul, deteriorating and full of symptoms (polluted oceans, ongoing wars, homeless people) that we need to 'get rid of'? He suggests that the decline in the quality of politics, of public debate and of public life is related to the Cartesian split: I am important, I am alive, it is important to 'go inside', work through my rages, become more whole: the world out there is 'dead', the world out there is secondary to me.

Hillman questions the assumption that rage, anger, heartbreak, are supposed to be 'processed' (ending up with what he calls 'processed psyche'). He questions, too, the uncovering of demons, quoting Rilke who said: 'I don't want the demons taken away because they're going to take my angels too' (Hillman and Ventura 1992, p.29). Wounds and scars, he says, are the stuff of character, are the stuff of art – the stuff that engages the imagination. Therapy (he rages) can make you boring: he talks of 'white bread' therapy honing away at the edges, removing the craziness, helping us to cope, to comply, to become 'good'. He urges us to be enraged and passionate about the world that we live in, for it too has 'soul', it too needs nurturing.

Perhaps, within this passionate discourse, rather than seeing music therapy as 'alleviating symptoms', we need to think in terms of intensifying them: invoking and evoking our passions, our rages and excitement, our madness; we need to think in terms of animating our total being, of quickening our spirit. We need therapy, perhaps, to awaken us from the psychic numbing that results from the condition that both Donald Winnicott, the psychoanalyst, and Michael Tippet, the composer, despair of: they mourn our lost passions. It seems that our creativity has been poured into machines, which now breathe and 'live' on our behalf.

If we reject the idea of symptoms and pathology, do we then need therapy? Do we need to be 'cured'? From what do we need 'curing'?

At the very least we know that we live in a collectively stressful, abrasive, ungentle world. We cannot remain separate from it. At the very least, we can say that therapy is a sanctuary: a place where we can stop, be still enough to hear and listen to other aspects of our lives, where we can see beyond the assault of information, and the distractions of (highly urbanised) life in the late 20th century. A place where somebody is there to assist the enlivening, the spiriting, the colouring, the meaning of life – meaning that we have successfully dispersed by collectively ditching our gods, our devils, our myths and our rituals. Indeed one of the delights of living in the African continent is that the 'ancestors', who exert powerful influences over daily life, thrive, both benevolently and malevolently.

Why Have Music Therapy?

The efficacy of music therapy for those who cannot speak, who have communication deficits, has been well enough documented, and is not the presiding focus here. However, what about music therapy for those of us who are high-functioning, verbally skilled, adept at making ourselves understood in our highly verbal mode? Do we want to subject ourselves to the baffling experience of therapy in another mode, a mode that is unfamiliar, that does not 'make sense', and that 'vanishes' after the session? If we want to work non-verbally, why not choose art therapy, where we can at least pin up the picture and live with it for a while? Why not have cognitive therapy, where we can name, target, plan, alter how we see the world and ourselves in it? Why not verbal psychotherapy, where, at least, we can 'hang on to' meaning?

Certainly, even in verbal psychotherapy, the experiencing of ourselves, through a language that has different nuances, can be a daunting, uncomfortable experience – and, of course, an exciting and illuminating one.

Even the shift from our native language to a foreign language – and all that this implies – is extremely complex in terms of our inner lives. Those of us who come from different linguistic backgrounds experience ourselves differently, in temperament and in concepts, depending on which language we speak. Eva Hoffman (1989) describes evocatively the loss of her sense of who she is, through the linguistic dispossession resulting from her family's emigration from Poland to Canada in the 1950s. She writes:

> The worst losses come at night… I wait for the spontaneous flow of inner language which used to be my night-time talk with myself, my way of informing the ego where the id had been. Nothing comes. Polish, in this short time, has atrophied, shrivelled from sheer

uselessness. Its words don't apply to my new experiences; they're not coeval with any of the objects, faces, or the very air I breathe in the daytime. In English, words have not penetrated to those layers of my psyche from which a private conversation could proceed... Now, this picture-and-word show is gone; the thread has snapped. I have no interior language, and without it, interior images – those images through which we assimilate the external world, through which we take it in, love it, make it our own – become blurred too. (pp.107, 108)

Is there a similarity of experience in clients who come to music therapy, 'sound' themselves through the medium of music? Here is a world that highlights and invites synchrony, multi-dimensions, space and time, simul-taneity – a world that has no access to sequential linearity, to linear logic and reason, a world that does not 'refer to', but that has its own interior laws, its own logic, a world that is itself. Like Eva Hoffman, do we, as clients, risk losing our familiar sense of self? Dare we risk finding another experience of ourselves?

My experience of work with verbal adults suggests that the experience of themselves through sound can be an epiphany: an illumination of recognising something new within something known. When Noel, whom we visited in Chapter 2, finished playing for the first time, he exclaimed with great vigour: 'this is me!! exactly!! this music that I just played!! I recognise this!'. This man recognised something about himself within moments of engaging in a different, and unfamiliar, medium, and was able in subsequent sessions to unravel and extend something about himself very quickly through the medium of music. Although he was sure that it was the fact that we worked through music that helped him, whereas months of (verbal) psycho-therapy had not come anywhere this near to addressing and identifying his issues, verbal psychotherapy may, in fact, have readied him for this experi-ence, by introducing him to a world in which the meaning of signs – of words – is not just limited and contained by the words themselves. In the same way the meaning of music was not just 'the music': its meaning was himself.

Ending and Beginning

This brief discussion has elicited issues that precede, in one sense, discourses about the inner workings of music therapy.

By choosing to work through the medium of music in music therapy – which in no sense dismisses or diminishes the value of using words – we remove ourselves from our more familiar mode, and immerse ourselves in the illusory, the immaterial, the intangible. All of these qualities risk being undervalued and dismissed by 'exterior' and rational psychological, medical and educational cultures, and in one sense, writing about music therapy is always a compromise in colour and focus.

Through music we attempt to repossess our imagination and, as Michael Tippett puts it, to regain our senses. Through music we can be cured from all the talking.

It seems that, as music therapists, we need to feel confident in the legitimacy of music as itself; of music as therapy; in the legitimacy of an intuition that is deliberate, and that will not be shrunk by compact definitions; and in the legitimacy of a self that is both healthy and ill, good and bad, moral and immoral, artistic and scientific. A self that is both verbal and musical. As music therapists we can allow ourselves, and one another, to be rooted in the 'medical' model, in the 'purely musical' model, in a 'psychodynamic' model – or to not be rooted at all. We may choose to ignore, or to draw from these and other discourses, as appropriate – with integrity. We can, perhaps, allow ourselves, and one another, to draw inspiration from Jung and from Freud, from the Dalai Lama and from Nelson Mandela, from Stravinsky and from Sting, without needing to defend, justify, deny or diminish one another's different perspectives. We can, however, insist on rigour – that does not narrow inspiration.

By allowing ourselves to shift from what James Hillman calls the 'numb insanity' of utterly sensible meaning and superb reasoning, towards the 'blessed madness' that allows meaning to be coloured by imagination and inexact rationality, we can enrich our understandings of Xolile, Noel, Jayne and Rose – and of ourselves. And we can be enriched by our authentic, and vulnerable, engagements with 'the world'.

I hope that the way music therapy has been explored in this book contributes to a less certain discourse, a less exact meaning, and to more musings.

References

Aiello, R. (ed) (1994) *Musical Perceptions.* Oxford: Oxford University Press.

Aigen, K. (1991) 'The roots of music therapy: towards an indigenous research paradigm.' Unpublished D. Arts Thesis, New York University.

Aigen, K. (1995) 'An aesthetic foundation of clinical theory: an underlying basis of creative music therapy.' In C.B. Kenny (ed) *Listening, Playing, Creating: Essays on the Power of Sound.* New York: State University of New York Press.

Aldridge, D. (1991) 'Aesthetics and the individual in the practice of medical research: discussion paper.' *Journal of the Royal Society of Medicine 84,* 147–150.

Aldridge, D. (1993a) 'Music therapy research II: research methods suitable for music therapy.' *The Arts in Psychotherapy 20,* 117–131.

Aldridge, D. (1993b) 'The music of the body: music therapy in medical settings.' *Journal of Mind-Body Health 9,* 1, 17–35.

Aldridge, D. and Aldridge, G. (1992) 'Two epistemologies: music therapy and medicine in the treatment of dementia.' *The Arts in Psychotherapy 19,* 243–255.

Aldridge, D. and Brandt, G. (1991) 'Music therapy and dementia.' *Journal of British Music Therapy 5,* 2, 28–36.

Aldridge, D., Brandt, G. and Wohler, D. (1990) 'Toward a common language among the creative art therapies.' *The Arts in Psychotherapy 17,* 189–195.

Alvarez, A. (1992) *Live Company: Psychoanalytic Psychotherapy with Autistic, Borderline, Deprived and Abused Children.* London: Tavistock/Routledge.

Ansdell, G. (1995) *Music For Life. Aspects of Creative Music with Adult Clients.* London: Jessica Kingsley Publishers.

Atik, Y. (1995) 'People factors in the performing arts.' *Performing Arts Medicine News 3,* 3, 7–12.

Baily, J. (1985) 'Music structure and human movement.' In P. Howell, I. Cross and R. West (eds) *Musical Structure and Cognition.* London: Academic Press.

Banister, P., Burman, E., Parker, I., Taylor, M. and Tindall, C. (1994) *Qualitative Methods in Psychology.* Open University Press.

Beebe, B. (1982) 'Micro-timing in mother–infant communication.' In M.R. Key (ed) *Nonverbal Communication Today.* New York: Mouton.

Beebe, B., Jaffe., Fedstein, S., Mays, K. and Alson, D. (1985) 'Interpersonal timing: the application of an adult dialogue model to mother–infant vocal and kinesic interactions.' In T.N. Field and N. Fox (eds) *Social Perception in Infants.* Norwood, N.J.: Ablex.

Bengtsson, I. and Gabrielsson, A. (1980) 'Methods for analyzing performance of musical rhythm.' *Scandinavian Journal of Psychology 21,* 257–268.

Bernieri, F.J. and Rosenthal, R. (1991) 'Interpersonal coordination: behavior matching and interactional synchrony.' In R.S. Feldman and B. Rime (eds) *Fundamentals of Nonverbal Behavior.* Cambridge University Press.

Bjorkvold, J.-R. (1992) *The Muse Within: Creativity and Communication, Song and Play from Childhood through Maturity.* New York: Harper Collins.

Blacking, J. (1973) *How Musical is Man?* London: Faber.

Blacking, J. (1987) *A Common-sense View of all Music.* Cambridge University Press.

Blacking, J. (1995) *Music, Culture, and Experience: Selected Papers.* Edited by R. Byron. Chicago: University of Chicago Press.

Bonny, H. (1978a) *Facilitating Guided Imagery and Music Sessions.* Monograph. Salina, Kansas: The Bonny Foundation.

Bonny, H. (1978b) *The Role of Taped Music Programs in the GIM Process.* Monograph No.2. Salina, Kansas: The Bonny Foundation.

Botez, M.I., Botez, T. and Aube, M. (1983) 'La neuromusicologie: partie integrante de la neuropsychologie clinique.' *L'union Medicale du Canada 112,* 4, 366–372.

Bowlby, J. (1969) *Attachment.* Penguin.

Brown, J.J. and Avsteieh, Z.A.K. (1989) 'On synchrony.' *The Arts in Psychotherapy 16,* 157–162.

Brown, S. (1992) 'Stretto: degrees of magnification.' *Journal of British Music Therapy 6,* 1, 21–22.

Brown, S. and Pavlicevic, M. (1996) 'Clinical improvisation in creative music therapy: musical aesthetic and the interpersonal dimension.' *The Arts in Psychotherapy 23,* 5, 397–406.

Bruscia, K. (1978) *Improvisional Models of Music Therapy.* St. Louis: Charles Thomas.

Bunt, L. (1994) *Music Therapy: An Art Beyond Words.* London: Routledge.

Bunt, L.G.K. and Hoskyns, S.L. (1987) 'A perspective on music therapy research in Great Britain.' *Journal of British Music Therapy 1,* 1, 4.

Burford, B. (1988) 'Action cycles: rhythmic actions for engagement with children and young adults with profound mental handicap.' *European Journal of Special Needs Education 3,* 4, 189–206.

Carter, A. (1992) Stretto. *Journal of British Music Therapy 6,* 1, 19.

Casement, P. (1985) *On Learning from the Patient.* Tavistock/Routledge.

Casement, P. (1988) *Further Learning from the Patient.* Routledge.

Chernoff, J.M. (1979) *African Rhythm and African Sensibility. Aesthetics and Social Action in African Musical Idioms.* Chicago: University of Chicago Press.

Christensen, A.L. (1974) *Luria's Neuropsychological Investigation (second edition).* Copenhagen: Munksgaard.

Clarke, E. (1988) 'Generative principles in music performance.' In J. Sloboda (ed) *Generative Processes in Music.* Oxford: Clarendon Press.

Condon, W.S. and Ogston, W.D. (1966) 'Sound film analysis of normal and pathological behaviour patterns.' *Journal of Nervous and Mental Diseases 143,* 4, 338–347.

Cook, N. (1990) *Music, Imagination, & Culture.* Oxford University Press.

Cook, N. (1994) 'Perception: a perspective from music theory.' In R. Aiello (ed) *Musical Perceptions*. Oxford University Press.

Copland, A. (1952) *Music and Imagination*. Cambridge University Press.

Cott, J. (1974) *Stockhausen: Conversations with the Composer*. Picador.

Dalhaus, C. (1989) *The Idea of Absolute Music*. Chicago: University of Chicago Press.

Davidson, J. (1996) 'The social in musical performance.' In D.J. Hargreaves and A. North (eds) *The Social Psychology of Music*. Oxford University Press.

Deutsch, D. (ed) (1982) *The Psychology of Music*. New York: Academic Press.

Dewey, J. (1934) *Art as Experience*. New York: Minton Balch.

Diaz de Chumaceiro, C.L. (1992) 'Transference countertransference in psychology integrations for music therapy in the 1970s and 1980s.' *Journal of Music Therapy XXIX*, 217–235.

Donald, M. (1991) *Origins of the Modern Mind: Three Stages in the Evolution of Culture and Cognition*. Cambridge, Massachusetts: Harvard University Press.

Dowling, W.J. and Harwood, D.L. (1986) *Music Cognition*. Orlando, Florida: Academic Press.

Feldstein, S. and Welkowitz, J.L. (1978) 'A chronography of conversation: in defense of an objective approach.' In A.W. Siegman and S. Feldstein (eds) *Nonverbal Behavior and Communication*. Hillsdale, NJ: Erlbaum.

Gabrielson, A. (1982) 'Perception and performance of musical rhythm.' In M. Clynes (ed) *Music, Mind, and Brain*. New York and London: Plenum Press.

Gale, C. (1992) Stretto. *Journal of British Music Therapy 6*, 2, 26.

Grout, D.J. (1960) *A History of Western Music*. London: Dent.

Guggenbuhl-Craig, A. (1971) *Power in the Helping Profession*. Dallas, Spring Publications.

Guntrip, H. (1971) *Psychoanalytic Theory, Therapy and the Self*. Basic Books.

Hanslick, E. (1957) *The Beautiful in Music*. New York: The Liberal Arts Press (transl. Gustav Cohen).

Hargreaves, D. (1986) *The Developmental Psychology of Music*. Cambridge: Cambridge University Press.

Hawkins, P. and Shohet, R. (1989) *Supervision in the Helping Professions*. OUP.

Heal, M. and Wigram, T. (ed) (1991) *Music Therapy in Health and Education*. London: Jessica Kingsley Publishers.

Hillman, J. (1975) *Re-Visioning Psychology*. Harper & Row.

Hillman, J. and Ventura, M. (1992) *We've had a Hundred Years of Psychotherapy and the World's Getting Worse*. San Francisco: Harper.

Hoffman, E. (1989) *Lost in Translation*. Minerva.

Howat, R. (1992) Stretto. *Journal of British Music Therapy 6*, 1, 22–23.

Howell, P., Cross, I., and West, R. (eds) (1985) *Musical Structure and Cognition*. London: Academic Press.

Hughes, M.H. (1995) 'A comparison of mother-infant interactions and the client-therapist realtionship in music therapy sessions.' In T. Wigram, B. Saperston and R. West (eds) *The Art and Science of Music Therapy: A Handbook*. Harwood Academic Publishers.

Humphrey, N. (1992) *A History of the Mind.* London: Vintage.

Illich, I. (1976) *Limits to Medicine.* Pelican.

John, D. (1995) 'The therapeutic relationship in music therapy as a tool in the treatment of psychosis.' In T. Wigram, B. Sapertson and R. West (eds) *The Art and Science of Music Therapy: A Handbook.* Harwood Academic Publishers.

Kandinsky, W. (1914) *Concerning the Spiritual in Art.* (1977 edition) New York: Dover Publications.

Karbusicky, V. (1987) 'The index sign in music.' *Semiotica 66,* 23–35.

Langer, S. (1951) *Philosophy in a New Key.* Mentor Books.

Lee, C. (1992) Stretto. *Journal of British Music Therapy 6,* 1, 23.

Lee, C.A. (1989) 'Structural analysis of therapeutic improvisatory music.' *Journal of British Music Therapy 3,* 2, 11–19.

Lee, C.S. (1985) 'The rhythmic interpretation of simple musical sequences: towards a perceptual model.' In P. Howell, I. Cross and R. West (eds) *Musical Structure and Cognition.* London: Academic Press.

Lee, C.S. (1991) 'The perception of metrical structure: experimental evidence and a model.' In P. Howell, R. West and I. Cross (eds) *Representing Musical Structure.* London: Academic Press.

Lerdahl, F. (1991) 'Underlying musical schemata.' In P. Howell, R. West and I. Cross (eds) *Representing Musical Structure.* London: Academic Press.

MacLaggan, D. (1994) 'The biter bit: subjective features of research in art and therapy.' In A. Gilroy and C. Lee (eds) *Art and Music: Therapy and Research.* London: Routledge.

Magee, W. (1995) 'Case studies in Huntington's Disease: music therapy assessment and treatment in the early to advanced stages.' *British Journal of Music Therapy 9,* 2, 13–19.

McDougall, J. (1993) 'Countertransference and primitive communication.' In A. Alexandris and G. Vaslamatzis (eds) *Countertransference Theory, Technique, Teaching.* London: Karnac Books.

McNamee, S. (1992) 'Reconstructing identity: the communal construction of crisis.' In S. McNamee and K.J. Gergen (eds) *Therapy as Social Construction.* Sage.

McNamee, S. and Gergen, K.J. (eds) (1992) *Therapy as Social Construction.* Sage.

Meyer, L. (1956) *Emotion and Meaning in Music.* Chicago: University of Chicago Press.

Meyer, L. (1967) *Music, The Arts and Ideas.* Chicago: University of Chicago Press.

Meyer, L. (1973) *Explaining Music.* Chicago: University of Chicago Press.

Meyer, L. (1994) 'Emotion and meaning in music.' In R. Aiello (ed) *Musical Perceptions.* Oxford University Press.

Milner, M. (1957) *On Not Being Able to Paint* (second edition). Heinemann.

Mitchell, S. (1993) *Hope and Dread in Psychoanalysis.* Basic Books.

Murray, L. (1988) 'Effects of postnatal depression on infant development: direct studies of early mother–infant interactions.' In I. Brockington and R. Kumar (eds) *Motherhood and Mental Illness 2.* Bristol: John Wright.

Murray, L. (1992) 'The impact of postnatal depression on infant development.' *Journal of Child Psychology and Psychiatry 33,* 3, 543–561.

Murray, L. and Stein, A. (1991) 'The effects of postnatal depression on mother–infant relations and infant development.' In M. Woodhead, R. Carr and P. Light (eds) *Becoming a Person*. London/New York: Routledge/Open University Press.

Murray, L. and Trevarthen, C. (1985) 'Emotional regulations of interactions between two-month-olds and their mothers.' In T.N. Field and N. Fox (eds) *Social Perception in Infants*. Norwood, N.J.: Ablex.

Murray, L. and Trevarthen, C. (1986) 'The infant's role in mother–infant communications.' *Journal of Child Language 13*, 15–29.

Nattiez, J.-J. (1990) *Music and Discourse: Towards a Semiology of Music*. Princeton University Press.

Neisser, U. (1976) *Cognition and Reality: Principles and Implications for Cognitive Psychology*. San Francisco: Fremans.

Nordoff, P. and Robbins, C. (1971) *Therapy in Music for Handicapped Children*. London: Gollancz.

Nordoff, P. and Robbins, C. (1977) *Creative Music Therapy*. New York: John Day.

Odell, H. (1989) 'Foreword.' *Journal of British Music Therapy 3*, 1, 3–4.

Oldfield, A. (1995) 'Communicating through music: The balance between following and initiating.' In T. Wigram, B. Saperston and R. West (eds) *The Art and Science of Music Therapy: A Handbook*. Harwood Academic Publishers.

Papousek, H. and Papousek, M. (1989) 'Forms and functions of vocal matching in interactions between mothers and their precanonical infants.' *First Language 9*, 137–158.

Papousek, M. (1996) 'Intuitive Parenting.' In I. Deliege and J. Sloboda (eds) *Musical Beginnings*. Oxford University Press.

Papousek, M. and Papousek, H. (1981) 'Musical elements in infants* vocalization: their significance for communication, cognition and creativity.' In L.P. Lipsitt (ed) *Advances in Infancy Research 1*. Norwood, N.J.: Ablex.

Papousek, M. and Papousek, H. (1991) 'The meanings of melodies in mothereses in tone and stress languages.' *Infant Behaviour and Development 14*, 415–440.

Papousek, M., Papousek, H. and Bornstein, M.H. (1985) 'The naturalistic vocal environment of young infants: on the significance of homogeneity and variability in parental speech.' In T.N. Field and N. Fox (eds) *Social Perception in Infants*. Norwood, N.J.: Ablex.

Papousek, M., Papousek, H. and Haekel, M. (1987) 'Didactic adjustments in fathers' and mothers' speech to their three-month-old infants.' *Journal of Psycholinguistic Research 16*, 491–516.

Pavlicevic, M. (1987) 'Reflections on the pre-musical moment.' *Journal of British Music Therapy 1*, 1, 22–24.

Pavlicevic, M. (1990) 'Dynamic interplay in clinical improvisation.' *Journal of British Music Therapy 4*, 2, 5–9.

Pavlicevic, M. (1991) 'Music in communication: improvisation in music therapy.' Unpublished PhD Thesis, University of Edinburgh.

Pavlicevic, M. (1994) 'Between chaos and creativity: music therapy with traumatised children in South Africa.' *British Journal of Music Therapy 8*, 2, 4–9.

Pavlicevic, M. (ed) (1995) *Forums '95.* Unpublished library monograph. Nordoff Robbins Music Therapy Centre.

Pavlicevic, M. (1995a) 'Interpersonal processes in clinical improvisation: towards a subjectively objective systematic definition.' In T. Wigram, B. Saperston and R. West (eds) *The Art and Science of Music Therapy: A Handbook.* Harwood Academic Publishers.

Pavlicevic, M. (1995b) 'Sounding into growth and growing into sound: improvisation groups with adults.' *The Arts in Psychotherapy 22,* 4, 359–367.

Pavlicevic, M. (1995c) 'Transforming a violent society.' *Human Development 16,* 2, 39–42.

Pavlicevic, M. (1996b) 'Music, meaning, and archaic forms.' *British Journal of Music Therapy 10,* 2, 14–20.

Pavlicevic, M. (1996a) 'Music-making in cross-cultural melt-down. Stretto.' *Journal of British Music Therapy 10,* 2, 34.

Pavlicevic, M. and Trevarthen, C. (1989) 'A musical assessment of psychiatric states in adults.' *Psychopathology 22,* 325–334.

Pavlicevic, M., Trevarthen, C. and Duncan, J. (1994) 'Music therapy and the rehabilitation of persons suffering from chronic schizophrenia.' *Journal of Music Therapy XXXI,* 2, 86–104.

Pressing, J. (1984) 'Cognitive processes in improvisation.' In W.R. Crozier and A.J. Chapman (eds) *Cognitive Processes in the Perception of Art.* Amsterdam: Elsevier.

Pribram, K.H. (1982) 'Brain mechanism in music.' In M. Clynes (ed) *Music, Mind, and Brain.* New York and London: Plenum Press.

Pierce, C. (1932) *Elements of Logic: Collected Papers, Vol. III.* C. Hartshorne and P. Weiss (eds) Cambridge, MA: Harvard University Press.

Priestley, M. (1975) *Music Therapy in Action.* New York: St. Martin's Press.

Priestley, M. (1988) 'Music and the Listeners.' *Journal of British Music Therapy 2,* 2, 9–13.

Robarts, J. (1994) 'Towards autonomy and a sense of self.' In D. Dokter (ed) *Arts Therapies and Clients with Eating Disorders.* London: Jessica Kingsley Publishers.

Robarts, J. (1996) 'Music therapy for children with autism.' In C. Trevarthen, K. Aitken, D. Papoudi and J. Robarts (eds) *Children with Autism.* London: Jessica Kingsley Publishers.

Roederer, J.G. (1982) 'Physical and neuropsychological foundations of music: the basic question.' In M. Clynes (ed) *Music, Mind, and Brain.* New York and London: Plenum Press.

Rogers, P. (1995) 'Music therapy research in Europe: a context for the qualitative/quantitative debate.' *Journal of British Music Therapy 9,* 2, 5–12.

Rose, G. (1992) *The Power of Form (expanded edition).* Madison, Conn.: International University Press.

Serafine, M.L. (1988) *Music as Cognition.* New York: Columbia University Press.

Shepherd, J. (1991) *Music as Social Text.* Cambridge: Polity Press.

Sloboda, J. (1985) *The Cognitive Psychology of Music.* Oxford University Press.

Sloboda, J., Davidson, J. and Howe, M. (1994) 'Is everyone musical?' *The Psychologist* 7, 7, 348–354.

Sobey, K. (1992) 'Stretto: the Relationship between music therapy and psychotherapy.' *Journal of British Music Therapy 6*, 1, 19–21.

Steiner, G. (1985) *Real Presences. The Leslie Stephen Memorial Lecture.* Cambridge University Press.

Stern, D. (1985) *The Interpersonal World of the Infant.* Basic Books.

Stern, D.N., Hofer, L., Haft, W. and Dore, J. (1985) 'Affect attunement: the sharing of feeling states between mother and infant by means of intermodal fluency.' In T.N. Field and N. Fox (eds) *Social Perception in Infants.* Norwood, N.J.: Ablex.

Stokes, M. (ed) (1994) *Ethnicity, Identity and Music.* Oxford, UK/Providence, USA: Berg.

Storr, A. (1972) *The Dynamics of Creation.* Harmondsworth: Penguin.

Stravinsky, I. (1974) *Poetics of Music.* Harvard University Press.

Streeter, E. (1987) 'Foreword.' *Journal of British Music Therapy 1*, 2, 3–5.

Streeter, E. (1995) Playing and talking: the dynamic relationship. Nordoff–Robbins International Symposium (tape recording of talk).

Sundberg, J. and Lindstrom, B. (1991) 'Generative theories for describing musical structure.' In P. Howell, R. West and I. Cross (eds) *Representing Musical Structure.* London: Academic Press..

Tippett, M. (1974) *Moving into Aquarius.* St Albans: Paladin.

Towse, E. (1991) 'Relationships in music therapy. Do music therapy techniques discourage the emergence of transference?' *British Journal of Psychotherapy 7*, 4, 323–330.

Trehub, S.E., and Trainor, L.J. (1993) 'Listening strategies in infancy: the roots of music and language development.' In S. McAdams and E. Brigand (eds) *Thinking in Sound: The Cognitive Psychology of Human Audition.* Oxford: Oxford University Press.

Trehub, S.E., Unyk, A.M. and Trainor, L.J. (1993a) 'Maternal singing in cross-cultural perspective.' *Infant Behaviour and Development 10*, 285–95.

Trehub, S.E., Unyk, A.M. and Trainor, L.J. (1993b) 'Adults identify infant-directed music across cultures.' *Infant Behaviour and Development 16*, 293–211.

Trevarthern, C. (1979) 'Communication and cooperation in early infancy. A description of primary intersubjectivity.' In M. Bullowa (ed) *Before Speech: The Beginning of Human Communication.* London: Cambridge University Press.

Trevarthen, C. (1980) 'The foundations of intersubjectivity: development of interpersonal and co-operative understanding in infants.' In D. Olson (ed) *The Social Foundations of Language and Thought: Essays in Honor of J.S. Bruner.* New York: W.W. Norton.

Trevarthen, C. (1986) 'Development of intersubjective motor control in infants.' In M.G. Wade and H.T.A. Whiting (eds) *Motor Development in Children: Aspects of Coordination and Control.* Dordrecht: Marthinus Nijhof, 209–261.

Trevarthen, C. (1987) 'Sharing makes sense: intersubjectivity and the making of an infant's meaning.' In R. Steele and T. Threadgold (eds) *Language Topics: Essays in Honor of Michael Halliday.* Amsterdam and Philadelphia: John Benjamins.

Trevathern, C. (1993) 'The self born in intersubjectivity: the psychology of an infant communicating.' In U. Neisser (ed) *Ecological and Interpersonal Knowledge of the Self.* New York: Cambridge University Press.

Trevarthen, C. and Aitken, K.J. (1994) 'Brain development, infant communication and empathy disorders: intrinsic factors in child mental health.' *Development and Psychopathology 6*, 599–635.

Tronik, E., Als, H. and Adamson, L. (1979) 'Structures of early face-to-face communicative interactions.' In M. Bullowa (ed) *Before Speech.* Cambridge: Cambridge University Press.

Unyk, A.M., Trehub, S.E., Trainor, L.J., and Schellenberg, E.G. (1992) 'Lullabies and simplicity: a cross-cultural perspective.' *Psychology of Music 20,* 15–28.

Vygotsky, L. (1986) *Thought and Language* (revised and edited by Alex Kozulin). Massachusetts Institute of Technology Press.

West, R., Howell, P. and Cross, I. (1985) 'Modelling perceived musical structure.' In P. Howell, I. Cross and R. West (eds) *Musical Structure and Cognition.* London: Academic Press.

West, R., Howell, P. and Cross, I. (1991) 'Musical structure and knowledge representation.' In P. Howell, R. West and I. Cross (eds) *Representing Musical Structure.* London: Academic Press.

Winnicott, D.W. (1971) *Playing and Reality.* Harmondsworth: Penguin.

Winnicott, D.W. (1988) *Human Nature.* Free Association Books.

Winnicott, D.W. (1990) The maturational process and the facilitating environment. Karnac.

Wheeler, B. (ed) (1995) *Music Therapy Research: Quantitative and Qualitative Perspectives.* Barcelona Publishers.

Yalom, I.D. (1989) *Love's Executioner and Other Tales of Psychotherapy.* Penguin Books.

Zohar, D. (1991) *The Quantum Self.* Flamingo.

Further Reading

Ansdell, G. (1996) 'Talking about music therapy: a dilemma and a qualitative experiment.' *British Journal of Music Therapy 10,* 1, 4–16.

Burman, E., Parker, I., Taylor, M. and Tindall, C. (1994) *Qualitative Methods in Psychology.* Open University Press.

Byron, R. (ed) (1995) *Music, Culture, & Experience.* Selected papers of John Blacking. Chicago: University of Chicago Press.

Gabrielsson, A. (1982) 'Perception of performance of musical rhythm.' In M. Clynes (ed) *Music, Mind and Brain: the Neuropsychology of Music.* New York and London: Plenum Press.

Index

Milton Keynes UK
Ingram Content Group UK Ltd.
UKHW032021121024
449584UK00006B/99